Critical Care Fo

8: Blood and Blood Tr

EDITOR
DR HELEN F GALLEY
Senior Lecturer in Anaesthesia and Intensive Care
University of Aberdeen

EDITORIAL BOARD
PROFESSOR NIGEL R WEBSTER
Professor of Anaesthesia and Intensive Care
University of Aberdeen

DR PAUL G P LAWLER
Clinical Director of Intensive Care
South Cleveland Hospital

DR NEIL SONI
Consultant in Anaesthesia and Intensive Care
Chelsea and Westminster Hospital

DR MERVYN SINGER
Reader in Intensive Care
University College Hospital, London

GALLEY

BMJ
Books

WO 480 H0204207

© BMJ Books 2002
BMJ Books is an imprint of the BMJ Publishing Group

First published in 2002
by BMJ Books, BMA House, Tavistock Square,
London WC1H 9JR

www.bmjbooks.com
www.ics.ac.uk

British Library Cataloguing in Publication Data

A catalogue record for this book is available from the British Library

ISBN 0-7279-1657-2

Typeset by Newgen Imaging Systems (P) Ltd, Chennai.
Printed and bound in Spain by GraphyCems, Navarra

Contents

Critical Care Focus series

Also available:

Contributors

Simon V Baudouin
Senior Lecturer in Intensive Care, University of Newcastle upon Tyne
Royal Victoria Infirmary, Newcastle upon Tyne, UK

Andrew Bodenham
Consultant in Anaesthesia & Intensive Care, Leeds General Infirmary, UK

Chris E Cooper
Professor of Biochemistry, Department of Biological Sciences, University
of Essex, Colchester, UK

Pierre-Francois Laterre
St Luc Hospital, Brussels, Belgium

Samuel J Machin
Consultant Haematologist, University College London Hospital, UK

Sheila MacLennan
Consultant in Transfusion Medicine, Leeds Blood Centre, UK

Claudio Martin
Associate Professor, London Health Sciences Centre, University of Western
Ontario, Canada

Hans J Nielson
Consultant Surgeon, Department of Surgical Gastroenterology,
Copenhagen University Hospital, Denmark

Martin G Tweeddale
Consultant in Intensive Care, Queen Alexandra Hospital, Portsmouth, UK

Preface to the Critical Care Focus series

The Critical Care Focus series aims to provide a snapshot of current thoughts and practice, by renowned experts. The complete series should provide a comprehensive guide for all health professionals on key issues in today's field of critical care. The volumes are deliberately concise and easy to read, designed to inform and provoke. Most chapters are produced from transcriptions of lectures given at the Intensive Care Society meetings and represent the views of world leaders in their fields.

Helen F Galley

Introduction

Transfusion requirements in critical care

Martin G Tweeddale

The art of fluid administration and haemodynamic support is one of the most challenging aspects of current critical care practice. Although more than half the patients in intensive care units receive blood transfusions there is little in the way of data to guide decisions on when to give transfusions. Despite published guidelines, based not on clinical trials, but on expert opinion, transfusion practice varies widely. Estimates of the frequency of inappropriate transfusion range from 4–66% in the literature. This article describes a multi-centre randomised controlled trial of a liberal versus a restrictive transfusion protocol in intensive care units in Canada. A transfusion strategy comprising a threshold of 70 g/l, with haemoglobin values maintained between 70 g/l and 90 g/l can be recommended in the light of this study, in stable resuscitated critically ill patients. This regime is both safe and cost-effective. Further research into blood product transfusion in critically ill patients should continue to be a priority, however.

Bioactive substances in blood for transfusion

Hans J Nielson

Transfusion associated acute reactions to allogeneic blood transfusions are frequent. In the surgical setting, peri-operative blood transfusion is related to both post-operative infectious complications and possibly predisposition to tumour recurrence in patients undergoing surgery for solid tumours. Removal of leucocytes by filtration may be of benefit, but some blood preparations are still detrimental. Pre-surgery deposition of autologous blood may be helpful, but only be of benefit in some types of surgery. This article presents the current state of transfusion-related post-operative complications.

Haemostatic problems in the intensive care unit

Samuel J Machin

Haemostatic failure is common in the intensive care unit. Haematological advice can, at times, be confusing, and therefore the remit of this article is to highlight specific areas of haemostatic failure, including both bleeding and thrombosis, that are relevant to patients on the intensive care unit. In addition, recent advances in terms of therapeutic strategies are discussed.

Activated protein C and severe sepsis

Pierre-Francois Laterre

The inflammatory and pro-coagulant host responses to infection are intricately linked. Decreased protein C levels observed in patients with sepsis are associated with increased mortality. This article briefly describes the interaction between inflammation and coagulation and the role of protein C in the regulation of this interaction. The results of a large multi-centre trial of activated protein C in patients with sepsis is also presented and discussed. Since reductions in the relative risk of death were observed regardless of whether patients had protein C deficiency at baseline, it is suggested that activated protein C has pharmacological effects beyond merely replacement of depleted endogenous levels. This observation suggests that measurements of protein C are not necessary to identify which patients would benefit from treatment with the drug.

Transfusion-related acute lung injury

Andrew Bodenham, Sheila MacLennan, Simon V Baudouin

Transfusion-related lung injury has been reported to occur in about 0·2% of all transfused patients, although it is thought that this may be an underestimate. The lung injury may be severe enough to warrant admission to the intensive care unit for ventilation, and is similar to acute respiratory distress syndrome in many respects. The exact cause of lung injury after transfusion remains confusing, although it is suggested to be due to the presence of donor antibodies. This article describes the clinical manifestations, possible causes and similarity to other lung conditions of transfusion-related lung injury and suggests future research strategies.

The use of colloids in the critically ill

Claudio Martin

Colloids are widely used in the replacement of fluid volume, although doubts remain as to their benefits. Different colloids vary in their molecular weight and therefore in the length of time they remain in the circulatory system. Because of this and their other characteristics, they may differ in their safety and efficacy. Plasma, albumin, synthetic colloids and crystalloids may all be used for volume expansion but the first two are expensive and crystalloids have to be given in much larger volumes than colloids to achieve the same effect. Synthetic colloids provide a cheaper, safe, effective alternative. There are three classes of synthetic colloid; dextrans, gelatins and hydroxyethyl starches; each is available in several formulations with different properties which affect their initial plasma expanding effects, retention in the circulation and side effects. This article describes the physiology of fluids and colloids, presents key animal studies that have contributed to the colloid-crystalloid debate, and describes the present clinical position.

Radical reactions of haem proteins

Chris E Cooper

This article provides an overview of basic free radical chemistry and biology before focusing on the reactions of haemoglobin and myoglobin as sources of free radical damage. Free radicals are implicated in many pathological conditions and free haem proteins in the circulation can participate in radical reactions which result in toxicity. These reactions have been shown to be relevant particularly in rhabdomyolysis and the side effects of haemoglobin-based blood substitutes. Clinical experience with chemically modified and genetically engineered haemoglobin blood substitutes have uncovered side effects that must be addressed before a viable oxygen-carrying alternative to blood can be developed. Research is now being directed towards understanding the mechanisms of these toxic side effects and developing methods of overcoming them.

1: Transfusion requirements in critical care

MARTIN G TWEEDDALE

On behalf of the Canadian Critical Care Trials Group and the Transfusion Requirements in Critical Care Investigators (PC Hebert, Principal Investigator, MA Blajchman, J Marshall, C Martin, G Pagliarello, I Schweitzer, MG Tweeddale and G Wells)

Introduction

The art of fluid administration and haemodynamic support is one of the most challenging aspects of current critical care practice. Although more than half the patients in intensive care units (ICU) receive blood transfusions there is little in the way of data to guide decisions on when to give transfusions. The American College of Physicians, among others, has published a transfusion algorithm.[1] However, this is based, not on controlled clinical trials, but on expert opinion. Despite these guidelines, transfusion practice varies widely. Estimates of the frequency of inappropriate transfusion range from 4–66% in the literature.[2] This article describes a multi-centre randomised controlled trial of a liberal versus a restrictive transfusion protocol in ICUs in Canada.[3] The trial was sponsored by the Canadian Critical Care Trials Group (an informal association of people interested in promoting critical care research) and was funded by the Canadian Medical Research Council and Bayer plc.

To transfuse or not to transfuse?

Prior to undertaking a clinical trial it is important to consider the arguments for and against treatment. Box 1.1 shows some reasons that doctors might give as to why stable patients in ICU should be transfused.

In fact, transfusion practice is a good example of how some patterns of treatment in critical care have been set prematurely without proper clinical or experimental evidence. The first four possibilities listed in Box 1.1 are each plausible, but none is proven or definitive. For example, it has been theorised that improving oxygen delivery and reducing oxygen debt would improve survival.[4] This has led to the assumption that transfusing patients on ICU is beneficial, with common practice dictating maintenance of haemoglobin concentrations at 100 or 120 g/l, despite some evidence of a detrimental effect of this practice.[5] Unfortunately, in Canadian critical

1

care units, less than 50% of blood transfusions are given for physiological reasons such as haemodynamic instability or active bleeding.[6] In effect, the majority of transfusions are given simply to achieve a specific laboratory value, and no specific change in physiological parameters is produced by the transfusion. This is confirmed by a recent study of blood transfusion practice in the London area.[7] This survey showed that 74% of the transfusions were given for "a low haemoglobin". In this survey the mean transfusion threshold was 88 g/l, but 25–30% of the transfusions were given at haemoglobin values above 90 g/l.

Box 1.1 Reasons for transfusing stable critically ill patients

- Augmenting oxygen delivery may improve outcome
- To decrease the risk of coronary ischaemia in coronary artery disease
- Age, disease severity and drugs may interfere with the normal adaptive response to anaemia
- To improve the "safety margin" in the event of further blood loss
- To achieve a specific laboratory value

If there are arguments for transfusion there are also arguments against. In Box 1.2, the first three statements are simply refutations of points made in Box 1.1 and like the latter, are plausible, but not properly substantiated. The first item in Box 1.2 illustrates a point which is often forgotten: physiological regulation is very effective, both in adapting to disease (such

---

Box 1.2 Reasons for not transfusing stable critically ill patients

- Red cell transfusions may not affect oxygen delivery
- Pathological supply dependency is rare
- No evidence that a higher haemoglobin concentration is of value in coronary artery disease
- Transfusion may impair microcirculation
- Transfusion may cause immunosuppression and increase infection rates
- The risks of transfusion may outweigh the benefits

---

as critical care anaemia) and in adapting to treatment (such as blood transfusion). For example, an increase in haemoglobin will almost certainly increase the oxygen carrying capacity of the blood. However, this may not necessarily increase oxygen delivery (unless this parameter is already inadequate). Rather, it is probable that cardiac output will fall to maintain the same oxygen delivery, but at a reduced level of cardiac work. In such a scenario, blood transfusion will not achieve the theoretical objective for which it was given.

The final three points in Box 1.2 do, however, raise substantive issues against unnecessary blood transfusion in critically ill patients. The penultimate point, in particular, is often ignored – among current critical care text books, only one mentions the possibility of immune consequences from blood transfusion, an issue addressed later in this volume (Chapter 2). It is indeed arguable that the risks of transfusion may outweigh the benefits.

Clinical trial

Existing practice before the trial

Before undertaking our trial of transfusion strategies, we surveyed more than 5000 patients admitted to six tertiary level ICUs in Canada, and found that 25% of patients received transfusions of red blood cells during the survey period.[6] Practice varied considerably, however, between ICUs, even after adjustment for patient age, acute physiological and chronic health evaluation (APACHE) II score, and diagnostic category. The most frequent reasons given for transfusing red blood cells were acute bleeding (35%) and augmentation of oxygen delivery (25%). The transfused patients received an average of 0·95 units per patient day. Given that 1650 patients were transfused, and that the average stay in ICU was approximately five days, this represents a very large amount of blood. Most (80%) of the transfusion orders were for two units, even though published guidelines suggest that only one unit should be transfused at a time. Figure 1.1 shows the mean transfusion thresholds for patients with low APACHE II scores (15 or below) in each of the six ICUs that were involved in the study.[6]

The transfusion threshold haemoglobin concentration varied from 79–95 g/l. In the UK the threshold haemoglobin level is similar to the mean value in the Canadian study, around 85–86 g/l, although the range goes from 78 g/l haemoglobin up to 95 g/l haemoglobin.[7] In another study, four specified scenarios were used as part of a national survey of Canadian critical care physicians.[8] Figure 1.2 shows that in the "trauma" scenario more than 50% of Canadian physicians would have accepted a haemoglobin of 85 g/l or less in their patient, but in a physiologically similar patient with active gastrointestinal bleeding, 50% of the physicians wanted

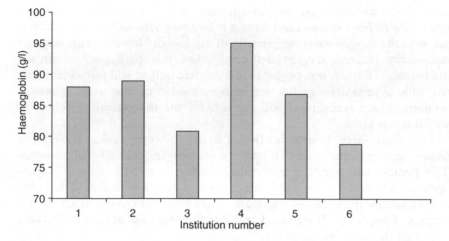

Figure 1.1 Mean transfusion thresholds by institution number in patients with APACHE II scores of 15 or less. Drawn, with permission, from data presented in Hebert PC, et al. Crit Care Med *1999;3:57–63.*[6]

to see a haemoglobin level of at least 100 g/l. This survey shows the marked differences in the approach of critical care doctors to transfusion in different clinical scenarios. This survey also found that >90% of Canadian critical care doctors would transfuse multiple units of red cells, despite guidelines to the contrary. Generally, practice varied widely between centres, physicians themselves, and patient groups.[6,8]

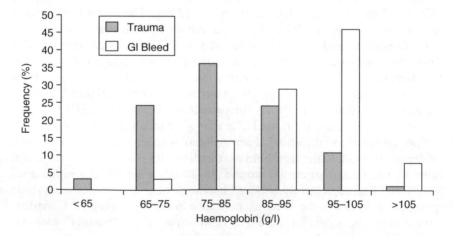

Figure 1.2 Transfusion thresholds in trauma and gastrointestinal bleed scenarios as identified by Canadian critical care physicians in a survey questionnaire. Drawn, with permission, from data presented in Hebert PC, et al. Crit Care Med *1999;3:57–63.*[6]

These studies[6,8] clearly showed that a state of "clinical equipoise" existed in the practice of transfusion in ICU, and that a randomised controlled trial was therefore warranted. The trial was titled "Transfusion Requirements in Critical Care" (TRICC). It was run from Ottawa with Paul Hebert as principal investigator, and an executive committee who reported regularly to the Canadian Critical Care Trials Group. The TRICC trial compared a restricted versus a liberal red cell transfusion strategy in terms of mortality and morbidity in adequately resuscitated critically ill patients.[3]

Study design

The study was randomised but could not be blinded. It was set up as an equivalency trial, powered to detect a 5% absolute difference in the primary end point (30-day all-cause mortality). Both type I and type II errors were set at 5%, and it was determined that 1620 patients were required. Twenty-five Canadian ICUs, 22 in University centres and 3 community ICUs, were involved in the study and, most importantly, the sub group analyses (APACHE II score above or below 20, and age above or below 55) were defined at the outset.

Any patient admitted to the ICU whose haemoglobin fell to 90 g/l or less within 72 hours was potentially eligible. Patients had to be adequately volume resuscitated, according to the discretion of the physicians, and the patients had to have a predicted length of ICU stay of at least another 24 hours. Obviously consent was also required. Exclusion criteria included pregnancy, age less than 16 years, and an inability to receive blood products. Patients who were actively bleeding (defined as a 30 g/l decrease in haemoglobin concentration or more than 3 units transfused over the preceding 12 hours) and patients with chronic anaemia (haemoglobin <90 g/l for more than 1 month previously) were also excluded. In addition, those with a hopeless prognosis or who were admitted for routine post-operative care after cardiac surgery were also excluded.

Study interventions

In patients randomised to the restrictive strategy, haemoglobin levels were maintained at 70–90 g/l with a transfusion trigger of 70 g/l. Those randomised to the liberal strategy had their haemoglobin concentrations maintained at 100–120 g/l, with a transfusion trigger of 100 g/l. The strategies were adhered to throughout the ICU stay but it was impractical to follow up beyond that. Patients received transfusions one unit at a time, with a subsequent check of the haemoglobin value. Other aspects of care were not controlled, but co-interventions were carefully monitored.

Results

Recruitment

A total of 6451 patients met the basic inclusion criterion, but only 838 were actually enrolled. This study therefore achieved only 52% of its target recruitment and was thus underpowered. The reasons why patients were missed or excluded are shown in Figure 1.3.

The TRICC trial suffered an unexpectedly high refusal rate (68%). The usual rate in Canada is about 45–50%. It was particularly concerning that about half the refusals were by the attending physicians rather than the patients or their relatives. This could potentially introduce bias into the

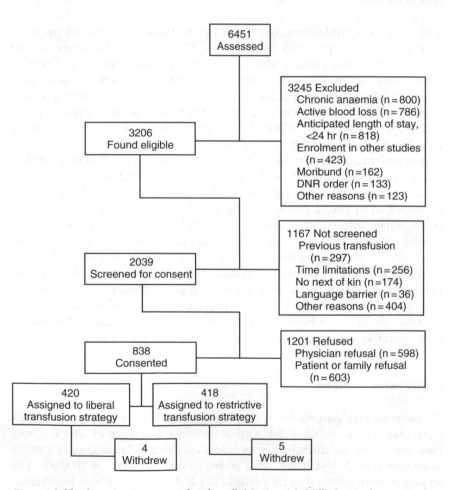

Figure 1.3 Numbers of patients assessed and enrolled in the trial. DNR denotes do not resuscitate. Previous transfusion indicates receipt of transfusion that increased the haemoglobin concentration to more than 90 g/l. Reproduced with permission from Hebert PC, et al. N Engl J Med 1999;340: 409–17.[3]

study, since the enrolled patients would not constitute a truly representative sample. However, in my own institution, the reasons why doctors refused consent for their patients were two-fold: half of them wanted their patients to receive blood and half of them did not. Clinical equipoise was thus eloquently demonstrated! Many family refusals were related to an unfortunate issue of timing. The study was run during a high profile national enquiry into administration of tainted blood involving threatened lawsuits and a great deal of media attention. Every time public awareness of the enquiry rose, recruitment went down, at least in this author's unit.

In the end 420 patients were randomised to the liberal strategy group and 418 to the restrictive strategy group. Fortunately there were very few withdrawals (see Figure 1.3).

Demographic data

The two groups were very well matched in terms of gender, age, APACHE II score and multiple organ dysfunction score at entry (Table 1.1). In terms of the ICU interventions patients were receiving on study entry, again the groups were also very well matched (Table 1.1). Pre-randomisation haemoglobin values, total fluid intake, the number of transfusions before

Table 1.1 Baseline characteristics of the two patient groups.

Patient characteristics	Liberal strategy group N = 420	Restrictive strategy group N = 418
Males (number)	255 (61%)	269 (64%)
Age (years)	58·1	57·0
APACHE II score	21·3	20·9
MODS	7·6	7·4
Mechanical ventilation (number)	346 (83%)	340 (82%)
Vascular catheter (number)	399 (95%)	393 (95%)
Pulmonary artery catheter (number)	150 (36%)	141 (34%)
Vasoactive drugs (number)	154 (37%)	153 (37%)
Patients on dialysis (number)	18 (4%)	21 (5%)
Surgical interventions (number)	17 (4%)	16 (4%)
Haemoglobin (g/dl)	8·2 ± 0·7	8·2 ± 0·7
Total fluid intake (l)	3·99 ± 1·71	3·95 ± 2·21
Tranfusions (units)	2·3 ± 4·6	2·5 ± 6·5
Lactate (mmol/l)	1·8 ± 2·1	1·8 ± 1·8

Data reproduced with permission from Hebert PC, *et al.* *N Engl J Med* 1999;**340**:409–17.[3]

enrolment and lactate concentrations were essentially identical in the two groups (Table 1.1).

Study intervention data

The mean haemoglobin concentrations after intervention were 107 g/l in the liberal strategy group and 85 g/l in the restrictive strategy group (p < 0·01). The number of units of blood transfused per patient was 5·2 units for the liberal group, and 2·5 units in the restricted group, a reduction of 54%. By protocol, all patients in the liberal group, and 33% of the restrictive group received no blood during their ICU stay. Compliance with the protocol was excellent (93% in the liberal group and 98% in the restrictive group) and there were very few crossovers (2·6% in the liberal group and 1% in the restrictive group).

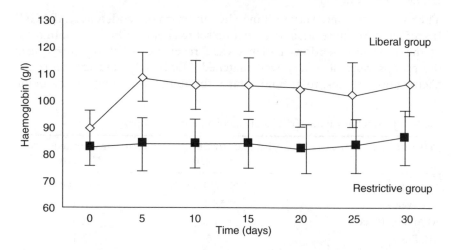

Figure 1.4 Haemoglobin concentration against days after admission to the intensive care unit in the restrictive strategy and liberal strategy groups in TRICC patients. Data are median and 95% confidence intervals. Drawn, with permission, from data presented in Hebert PC, et al. N Engl J Med 1999;340:409–17.[3]

Figure 1.4 shows haemoglobin values plotted against time. In the restrictive group a relatively steady value with a constant error was seen. In the liberal strategy group values decreased slightly over time and the error bars became wider. However the haemoglobin values were statistically significantly different at all time points between the two groups.

All cause 30-day mortality was 23·3% (98 patients died) in the liberal strategy group and 18·7% (78 patients died) in the restrictive strategy group – an absolute difference of 5%. However, due to low recruitment to the study, this difference failed to reach significance (p = 0·11). There were no significant differences between the groups in ICU stay or organ dysfunction scores. Thus, at the very least, the TRICC trial shows that there is no clinical advantage in transfusing resuscitated ICU patients to haemoglobin values above 70–90 g/l. Furthermore, such a restrictive transfusion policy is associated with a considerable reduction in the amount of blood used.

While the overall results failed to show a significant difference between the two transfusion strategies, the pre-determined sub-group analyses were very revealing. In the patients with an APACHE II score <20, 30-day all-cause mortality was 8·7% in the conservative strategy patients, compared to 16·1% in the liberal strategy patients (p = 0·02). In the patients with APACHE II scores of >20, there was no difference in mortality (31% in the liberal group and 28·3% in the restrictive group). Similarly, in younger patients (but not in those over 55 years of age) there was a statistically significant mortality difference that favoured the restricted strategy. Figure 1.5

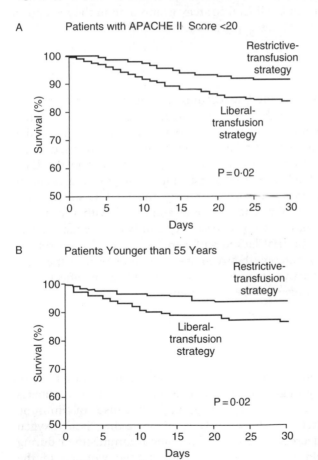

Figure 1.5 Kaplan-Meier estimates of survival in patients: A. with APACHE II scores below 20 and B. aged below 55 years. Reproduced with permission from Hebert PC, et al. N Engl J Med 1999;340:409–17.[3]

shows the Kaplan-Meier survival curves for the patients sub-grouped according to APACHE II score or age. It can be seen that the significant mortality advantage of the restrictive transfusion strategy in patients with APACHE II scores below 20, or aged below 55 years, is apparent immediately and is held throughout the study period. We can conclude that unnecessary transfusions in younger, less sick patients in ICU are actually harmful.

Complications

Cardiac complications were more common in the liberal strategy group (21% versus 13%, $p < 0.01$). There were differences in the number of new infarctions (12 versus 3 cases; $p < 0.02$) and pulmonary oedema (45 versus 22 cases; $p < 0.01$). Acute respiratory distress syndrome showed a tendency to occur more frequently in the liberal strategy group than in the restrictive strategy group (48 versus 32 cases; $p = 0.06$).

Summary

The TRICC trial, although limited by recruitment difficulties, was well-run with >93% compliance with the protocol, and few crossovers. Within the restrictive group, red blood cell transfusion use was reduced by 54% and a third of the patients randomised to this group were not transfused at all during their ICU stay. With an average cost of £72 per unit in the UK, introduction of the TRICC restrictive transfusion strategy would result in very substantial savings in blood costs. Similarly, the TRICC strategy has advantages of cost, practicality and outcome compared with the use of erythropoietin, which has been proposed to combat anaemia in the critically ill.[9] Although the trial lacked sufficient power to demonstrate a significant difference in outcome between the two strategies, in the sub-group analysis the restrictive strategy was significantly more effective in terms of mortality in younger and less ill patients.

Conclusion

The TRICC trial has added to the literature showing harmful effects of blood transfusion. Why might this be so? The blood given in the liberal transfusion strategy may be harmful perhaps because of immune suppression (see Chapter 2). Alternatively, it might be that tissue oxygen delivery was actually decreased. Much of the blood administered during the TRICC trial would be old (>16days) due to the working of the Canadian Blood Transfusion Service. The age of blood may have significant effects on clinical outcome.[10] Since old blood is non-deformable, it can clog capillaries, and this may be particularly relevant in septic patients who already have microvascular abnormalities. Thus tissue oxygen delivery may be actually decreased even though haemoglobin is increased.[11] The presence and non-reversibility of storage lesions in old blood is well known and may have contributed to the adverse consequences documented in the TRICC trial. On the other hand, the beneficial effects of the restrictive strategy may arise from haemodilution, reducing blood viscosity and so promoting oxygen delivery and improving flow in the microcirculation. These points reiterate that we know very little about this product which we give so freely to our critically ill patients.

No study is perfect and this one was no exception. The study was underpowered due to high refusal rates from physicians and relatives. Whilst it is possible that this may have introduced bias in the selection of patients for the study, there is no evidence to support this. The patients enrolled do seem to represent a broad range of typical ICU patients and therefore the trial results should be generally applicable, including patients admitted to critical care units with various primary or secondary cardiovascular diagnoses.[12] The one exception which should be noted is that patients with acute coronary syndromes were very uncommon in our study population because in Canada (as in the UK), most of these patients are admitted to cardiac care units rather than ICU. It therefore remains possible that the TRICC trial results would not be applicable to this patient group.

Leucocyte depleted blood is now available in the UK and in Canada and its use might ameliorate the harmful effects of the liberal strategy. But one should ask why blood should be given at £72 per unit when no clinical benefit would be expected? The TRICC trial clearly shows that stable resuscitated critically ill patients do very well if they are maintained with haemoglobin values of 70–90 g/l.

There are two recommendations which are applicable in the light of this study. In stable, resuscitated, critically ill patients, a transfusion strategy comprising a threshold of 70 g/l, with haemoglobin values maintained between 70–90 g/l should normally be used. This regime is both safe and cost-effective. Secondly, further research into blood product transfusion in ICU patients should be a priority for the critical care community.

References

1 American College of Physicians. Practice strategies for elective red blood cell transfusion. *Ann Intern Med* 1992;**116**:403–6.
2 Hebert PC, Schweitzer I, Calder L, Blajchman M, Giulivi A. Review of the clinical practice literature on allogeneic red blood cell transfusion. *Can Med Assoc J* 1997;**156**:S9–S26.
3 Hebert PC, Wells G, Blajchman MA, *et al.* A multicenter, randomized, controlled clinical trial of transfusion requirements in critical care. Transfusion Requirements in Critical Care Investigators, Canadian Critical Care Trials Group. *N Engl J Med* 1999;**340**:409–17.

4   Shoemaker WC, Appel PL, Kram HB, Waxman K, Lee TS. Prospective trial of supranormal values of survivors as therapeutic goals in high-risk surgical patients. *Chest* 1988;**94**:1176–86.
5   Boyd O, Grounds RM, Bennett ED. A randomized clinical trial of the effect of deliberate perioperative increase of oxygen delivery on mortality in high-risk surgical patients. *JAMA* 1993;**270**:2699–707.
6   Hebert PC, Wells G, Martin C, *et al.* Variation in red cell transfusion practice in the intensive care unit: a multi-centre cohort study. *Crit Care Med* 1999;**3**:57–63.
7   Boralessa H, Rao M, Soni N, *et al.* Blood and component use in intensive care. *Br J Anaesth* 2001;**87**:347P(abstract).
8   Hebert PC, Wells G, Martin C, *et al.* A Canadian survey of transfusion practices in critically ill patients. Transfusion Requirements in Critical Care Investigators and the Canadian Critical Care Trials Group. *Crit Care Med* 1998;**26**:482–7.
9   Corwin HL, Gettinger A, Rodriguez RM, *et al.* Efficacy of recombinant human erythropoietin in the critically ill patient: A randomised, double-blind, placebo-controlled trial. *Crit Care Med* 1999;**27**:2346–50.
10 Purdy FR, Tweeddale MG, Merrick PM. Association of mortality with age of blood transfused in septic ICU patients. *Can J Anaesth* 1997;**44**:1256–61.
11 Marik PE, Sibbald WJ. Effect of stored-blood transfusion on oxygen delivery in patients with sepsis. *JAMA* 1993;**21**:3024–29.
12 Hebert PC, Yetisir E, Martin C, Blajchman MA, Wells G, Marshall J, Tweeddale M, Pagliarello G, Schweitzer I. Is a low transfusion threshold safe in critically ill patients with cardiovascular diseases? *Crit Care Med* 2001;**29**:227–34.

2: Bioactive substances in blood for transfusion

HANS J NIELSEN

Introduction

Transfusion associated acute reactions to allogeneic blood transfusions are frequent. In the surgical setting, peri-operative blood transfusion is related to both post-operative infectious complications and possibly pre-disposition to tumour recurrence in patients undergoing surgery for solid tumours. Removal of leucocytes by filtration may be of benefit, but some blood preparations are still detrimental. Pre-surgery deposition of autologous blood may be helpful, but only be of benefit in some types of surgery. This article will present the current state of transfusion related post-operative complications.

Blood transfusion – what do we mean?

The issue of side effects of blood transfusion has to be considered in the context of the different blood products currently available for transfusion: for example there are the allogeneic blood components – either leucodepleted or not, at the bedside or before storage, but in addition, autologous blood components can be transfused, from sources including pre-operative donation, acute normovolaemic haemodilution, intra-operative salvage and post-operative drainage. More recently, artificial oxygen carriers such as crosslinked haemoglobins may be relevant. It is important when looking at specific reports concerning side effects of blood transfusion to realise what was actually given to the patient.

Infection after surgery

There are also several factors that can contribute to the complications after surgery, which might cloud the interpretation on the effects of transfusion. Patients undergoing intra-abdominal surgery have a high risk of developing post-operative infectious complications, from bacterial contamination, the immune status and also the environment. Impaired immunity pre-operatively

13

can be mediated through several mechanisms, including the presence of solid tumours, the nutritional state of the patient (see *Critical Care Focus*, Volume 7), whether patients have pre-existing infections, the presence of large bowel perforation or indeed, long standing alcohol abuse.[1] Post-operatively, development of infectious complications can rapidly overwhelm the patient's immune defences, pre-disposing to further infection.

Infectious complications and blood transfusion

The frequency of post-operative infectious complications is significantly increased in patients with colorectal cancer receiving peri-operative blood transfusion. In a study by Mynster *et al*,[2] patient risk variables, variables related to operation technique, blood transfusion and the development of infectious complications were recorded prospectively in 740 patients undergoing elective resection for primary colorectal cancer. The patients were analysed in four groups depending on whether or not they received peri-operative blood transfusions and whether post-operative infectious complications developed. There were less infectious complications in the non-transfused compared to the transfused patients (19% and 31% respectively) and multivariate analysis showed that risk of death was significantly increased in patients who developed infection after transfusion compared with patients receiving neither blood transfusion nor developing infection. This is elegantly demonstrated in Figure 2.1. The authors concluded that blood transfusion *per se* may not be a risk factor for poor prognosis after colorectal cancer surgery, but the combination of peri-operative blood transfusion and subsequent development of post-operative infectious complications may be associated with a poor prognosis.

To determine whether blood transfusion influences infection after trauma, Agarwal and co-workers[3] analysed data from 5366 consecutive patients hospitalised for more than 2 days following severe trauma. The incidence of infection was significantly related to the mechanism of injury. Stepwise logistic regression analyses of infection showed that the amount of blood received and the Injury Severity Score were the only two variables that were significant predictors of infection. Even when patients were stratified by Injury Severity Score, the infection rate increased significantly with increases in the numbers of units of blood transfused. This study revealed that in trauma as well as in patients undergoing surgery for cancer, blood transfusion is an important independent statistical predictor of infection and this effect is unattributable to age, sex, or the underlying mechanism of injury.

In patients undergoing hip replacement surgery, the infectious complication rate is extremely low – around 5%. This is surgery that has an inherently low risk of bacterial contamination. A retrospective review[4] of patients undergoing orthopaedic surgery compared the rate of the post-operative infectious

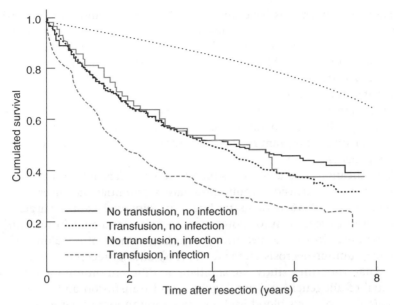

Figure 2.1 Kaplain-Meier analysis of survival in patients with colorectal cancer. P = 0·0001 between the four groups (Log rank test). The upper dotted line represents the overall survival of a cohort of parish inhabitants with the same age and sex distribution as the study populations. Reproduced from Mynster T, et al. Br J Surg 2000;87:1553–62[2] with permission.

complications in patients receiving allogeneic transfusion, autologous transfusion, both types, or no transfusion. The overall post-operative infection rate was 6·1% and was similar in those receiving allogeneic, autologous or both types of transfusion. Among those patients who received allogeneic transfusions, a subset of 15 patients received whole blood transfusions and had an infection rate of 20%. Significant predictors of post-operative infection included increasing age, spinal surgery, high admission haematocrit, and greater time in surgery. Only the use of allogeneic whole blood was a significant predictor of post-operative infection, which suggests a detrimental effect of allogeneic plasma.

However, in patients undergoing elective operations for colorectal cancer, transfusion of autologous blood was associated with significantly fewer post-operative infective complications than transfusion of allogeneic blood or no blood transfusion.[5]

Tumour recurrence and transfusion

The study by Mynster[2] et al. described above shows that blood transfusion alone does not affect long term survival or recurrence of disease. This is seen in Figure 2.1, where the survival curves for transfusion and no infection are the same as no transfusion and no infection. However patients who receive blood transfusion and subsequently develop post-operative infectious complications have much higher mortality and a greater risk of disease recurrence. The immunosuppressive effect of allogeneic blood transfusions can be associated with a poor prognosis for cancer patients. Pre-deposit autologous blood transfusions could be a solution to overcome this putative deleterious effect. In a randomised study[6] to compare the effects of autologous with allogeneic blood transfusions in colorectal cancer patients, there was no significant difference in disease-free survival between both groups. It was concluded that the use of a pre-deposit autologous blood transfusion programme does not improve the prognosis in colorectal cancer patients.

The indications that autologous blood transfusion is not immunologically neutral but has intrinsic immunomodulatory potential was investigated in another study[7] of 56 patients undergoing colorectal cancer surgery and randomised to receive autologous or allogeneic blood transfusion. Various immune mediators were measured, including soluble interleukin-2 (IL-2) receptor, tumour necrosis factor α (TNFα) and its receptors, and IL-10. The data from this study substantiate a different immunomodulatory potential of allogeneic and autologous blood transfusion and suggest that transfused autologous blood itself exerts an immunomodulatory effect.

These studies, which indicate an immune effect even from autologous blood transfusion in patients undergoing surgery for colorectal cancer, suggest that there is a common factor present in both types of blood transfusion that is exerting this effect.

Vascular endothelial growth factor and metastases

The ability of a tumour to metastasise is related to the degree of angiogenesis it induces. In addition, micrometastases rely on new vessel formation to provide the nutrients necessary for growth.[8] Angiogenesis is therefore decisive in tumour progression and metastasis. Vascular endothelial growth factor (VEGF) is a potent angiogenic factor. In the study by Werther and colleagues,[9] it was shown that patients with colorectal cancer had significantly higher levels of soluble circulating VEGF, compared to healthy blood donors, and levels were related to cancer staging. In conclusion, this study suggested a biological significance of VEGF in patients with colorectal cancer. In some patients with lung cancer, secondary lung metastasis appears soon after pulmonary surgery such that post-operative weakness of tumor angiogenesis suppression mechanisms seems to play an important role in the recurrence of lung metastases. Serum VEGF increased after pulmonary surgery and *in vitro* studies showed that VEGF played an important role in the rapid growth of dormant micrometastases of the lung. This study suggested that the post-operative increases in VEGF disrupted angiogenesis suppression and induced the growth of dormant micrometastases early in the post-operative period.[10] These studies then lead to speculation that VEGF was released during storage of blood, which when transfused during surgery in patients with cancer, was leading to stimulation of angiogenesis and tumour growth.

The effects of storage

Reduced survival after curative surgery for solid tumours may therefore be linked to blood transfusion as a result of cancer growth factors present in transfusion components. In a study by this author,[11] VEGF was measured in serum and plasma samples and in lysed cells from healthy volunteers and in non-filtered and pre-storage white cell-reduced whole blood, buffy coat-depleted saline-adenine-glucose-mannitol (SAGM) blood, platelet-rich plasma, and buffy coat-derived platelet pools obtained from volunteer, healthy blood donors. The extracellular accumulation of VEGF was also determined in non-filtered white cell-reduced and SAGM blood during storage for 35 days and in buffy coat derived platelet pools during storage for 7 days. VEGF accumulated significantly in various blood fractions depending on the storage time. The accumulation of VEGF was high enough to stimulate cancer growth in animals when we transfuse not only red cells in non-leucodepleted blood but also cancer promoting substances.

Other leucocyte- and platelet-derived bioactive mediators are also released during storage of various blood components for transfusion, including eosinophil cationic protein, eosinophil protein X, myeloperoxidase and plasminogen activator inhibitor-1[12] (Figure 2.2).

Leucofiltration

Removal of leucocytes from allogeneic blood transfusions has been suggested to reduce release of bioactive substances compared to non-filtered whole blood. In a study[13] of colorectal cancer patients undergoing surgery, transfusion with whole blood induced a significant decrease in lymphocyte proliferation and a significant increase in soluble IL-2 receptor and IL-6 levels. In patients transfused with leucocyte-depleted blood only slight and transient changes were observed, which were not significantly different from those observed in non-transfused patients. Cell-mediated immunity, assessed by skin testing with seven common delayed-type hypersensitivity antigens, was also depressed to a greater extent in patients who received whole blood than in those who received filtered blood or who did not receive a blood transfusion.[14] The effect of pre-storage versus bedside-leucofiltration on reduction of bioactive substances and leucocyte content in donor blood was studied by Hammer et al.[15] Extracellular release of content of myeloperoxidase, eosinophil cationic protein, histamine and plasminogen activator inhibitor-1 were reduced in blood which was filtered before storage (Figure 2.3).

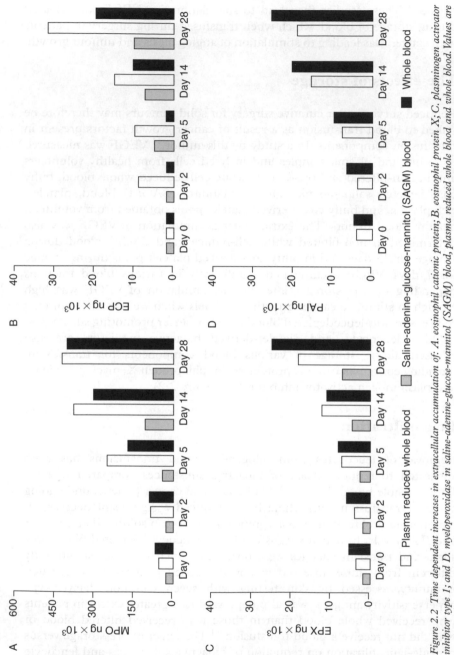

Figure 2.2 Time dependent increases in extracellular accumulation of: A. eosinophil cationic protein; B. eosinophil protein X; C. plasminogen activator inhibitor type 1; and D. myeloperoxidase in saline-adenine-glucose-mannitol (SAGM) blood, plasma reduced whole blood and whole blood. Values are medians. Asterisk indicates p < 0·05 for plasma reduced whole blood compared to SAGM blood and whole blood. Reproduced from Nielsen HJ, et al. Transfusion 1996;**36**:960–5[12] with permission.

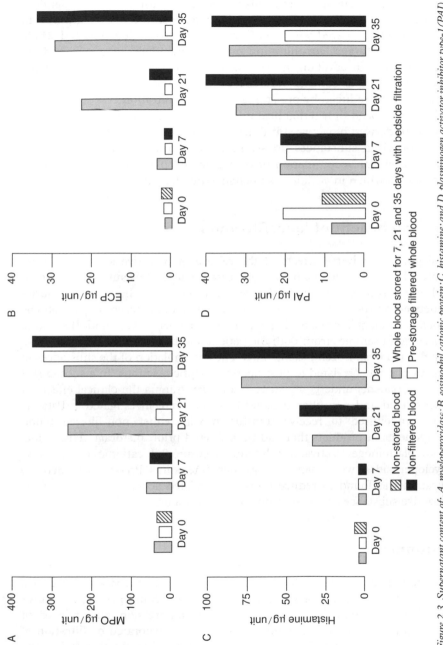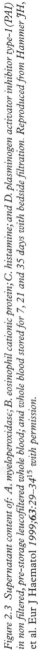

*Figure 2.3 Supernatant content of: A. myeloperoxidase; B. eosinophil cationic protein; C. histamine; and D. plasminogen activator inhibitor type-1 (PAI) in non filtered, pre-storage leucofiltered whole blood; and whole blood stored for 7, 21 and 35 days with bedside filtration. Reproduced from Hammer JH, et al. Eur J Haematol 1999;**63**:29–34[15] with permission.*

Pre-storage leucofiltration also reduced storage-time-dependent suppression of *in vitro* stimulated TNFα release induced by plasma from whole blood compared with non-filtered and bedside-leucofiltered whole blood.[16] Pre-storage leucofiltration may thus be advantageous to bedside leucofiltration. In addition, fresh frozen plasma prepared by conventional separation methods contains various leucocyte-derived bioactive substances, which may be reduced by pre-storage leucocyte filtration.[17]

It has also been shown that heating reduces accumulation of extracellular leucocyte-derived bioactive substances in whole blood, whereas it increases platelet-derived substances. Pre-storage leucofiltration, however, reduces the extracellular accumulation of leucocyte and platelet-derived bioactive substances, which in addition is unchanged by heating.[18]

Clinical benefit of leucofiltration

The potential adverse effects of the release of bioactive substances were analysed in a burn trauma patient in a case report by this author.[19] A patient with 40% second and third degree burn trauma without other injuries underwent a two-step transplantation operation. Histamine, eosinophil cationic protein, eosinophil protein X, neutrophil myeloperoxidase and IL-6 were measured in samples from both the patient and from all transfused red cell, platelet and fresh frozen plasma units. The accumulation of the substances in patient plasma correlated to post-operative septic reactions. In a subsequent study of patients undergoing surgery for burn trauma the clinical effects of leucofiltered and non-filtered blood products were investigated.[20] Patients were randomised to receive transfusion with either non-filtered blood components or products that had been filtered prior to storage. Histamine, IL-6, plasminogen activator inhibitor-1, eosinophil cationic protein and myeloperoxidase were analysed at various time points. Pre-storage leucocyte filtration was found to reduce transfusion related accumulation of various bioactive substances in burn trauma patients (Figure 2.4).

Summary

Peri-operative allogeneic blood transfusion increases the risk of infectious complications after major surgery and of cancer recurrence after curative operation and may be related to immunosuppression and release of angiogenic mediators. These effects seem to be ameliorated by filtration of blood prior to storage. The use of autologous blood might also reduce the detrimental effects of transfusion, but studies have unexpectedly shown similar post-operative infectious complications and cancer recurrence and/or survival rates in patients receiving autologous blood donated before operation and in those receiving allogeneic blood.

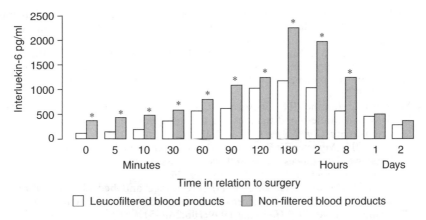

Figure 2.4 Serum concentrations of interleukin-6 in patients undergoing surgery for burn trauma and randomised to received either pre-storage leucofiltered blood components or non-filtered components. Values are median. Asterisk indicates p < 0·05 between groups. Reproduced from Nielsen HJ, et al. Burns 1999;25:162–70[20] with permission.

References

1   Nielsen HJ. The effect of histamine type-2 receptor antagonists on posttraumatic immune competence. *Dan Med Bull* 1995;**42**:162–74.

2   Mynster T, Christensen IJ, Moesgaard F, Nielsen HJ. Effects of the combination of blood transfusion and postoperative infectious complications on prognosis after surgery for colorectal cancer. Danish RANX05 Colorectal Cancer Study Group. *Br J Surg* 2000;**87**:1553–62.

3   Agarwal N, Murphy JG, Cayten CG, Stahl WM. Blood transfusion increases the risk of infection after trauma. *Arch Surg* 1993;**128**:171–6.

4   Fernandez MC, Gottlieb M, Menitove JE. Blood transfusion and postoperative infection in orthopedic patients. *Transfusion* 1992;**32**:318–22.

5   Vignali A, Braga M, Dionigi P, *et al.* Impact of a programme of autologous blood donation on the incidence of infection in patients with colorectal cancer. *Eur J Surg* 1995;**161**:487–92.

6   Busch OR, Hop WC, Marquet RL, Jeekel J. The effect of blood transfusions on survival after surgery for colorectal cancer. *Eur J Cancer* 1995;**31A**:1226–8.

7   Heiss MM, Fraunberger P, Delanoff C, *et al.* Modulation of immune response by blood transfusion: evidence for a differential effect of allogeneic and autologous blood in colorectal cancer surgery. *Shock* 1997;**8**:402–8.

8   McNamara DA, Harmey JH, Walsh TN, Redmond HP, Bouchier-Hayes DJ. Significance of angiogenesis in cancer therapy. *Br J Surg* 1998;**85**:1044–55.

9   Werther K, Christensen IJ, Brunner N, Nielsen HJ. Soluble vascular endothelial growth factor levels in patients with primary colorectal carcinoma. The Danish RANX05 Colorectal Cancer Study Group. *Eur J Surg Oncol* 2000;**26**:657–62.

10 Maniwa Y, Okada M, Ishii N, Kiyooka K. Vascular endothelial growth factor increased by pulmonary surgery accelerates the growth of micrometastases in metastatic lung cancer. *Chest* 1998;**114**:1668–75.

11 Nielsen HJ, Werther K, Mynster T, Brunner N. Soluble vascular endothelial growth factor in various blood transfusion components. *Transfusion* 1999;**39**:1078–83.

12 Nielsen HJ, Reimert CM, Pedersen AN, *et al*. Time-dependent, spontaneous release of white cell- and platelet-derived bioactive substances from stored human blood. *Transfusion* 1996;**36**:960–5.
13 Jensen LS, Hokland M, Nielsen HJ. A randomized controlled study of the effect of bedside leucocyte depletion on the immunosuppressive effect of whole blood transfusion in patients undergoing elective colorectal surgery. *Br J Surg* 1996;**83**:973–7.
14 Nielsen HJ, Hammer JH, Moesgaard F, Kehlet H. Comparison of the effects of SAG-M and whole-blood transfusions on postoperative suppression of delayed hypersensitivity. *Can J Surg* 1991;**34**:146–50.
15 Hammer JH, Mynster T, Reimert CM, Pedersen AN, Nielsen HJ. Reduction of bioactive substances in stored donor blood: prestorage versus bedside leucofiltration. *Eur J Haematol* 1999;**63**:29–34.
16 Mynster T, Hammer JH, Nielsen HJ. Prestorage and bedside leucofiltration of whole blood modulates storage-time-dependent suppression of *in vitro* TNFalpha release. *Br J Haematol* 1999;**106**:248–51.
17 Nielsen HJ, Reimert C, Pedersen AN, *et al*. Leucocyte-derived bioactive substances in fresh frozen plasma. *Br J Anaesth* 1997;**78**:548–52.
18 Hammer JH, Mynster T, Reimert CM, *et al*. Effect of heating on extracellular bioactive substances in stored human blood: *in vitro* study. *J Trauma* 1997;**43**:799–803.
19 Nielsen HJ, Reimert CM, Dybkjaer E, Roed J, Alsbjorn B. Bioactive substance accumulation and septic complications in a burn trauma patient: effect of perioperative blood transfusion. *Burns* 1997;**23**:59–63.
20 Nielsen HJ, Hammer JH, Krarup AL, *et al*. Prestorage leukocyte filtration may reduce leukocyte-derived bioactive substance accumulation in patients operated for burn trauma. *Burns* 1999;**25**:162–70.

3: Haemostatic problems in the intensive care unit

SAMUEL J MACHIN

Introduction

Haemostatic failure is common in the intensive care unit (ICU). Haematological advice can, at times, be confusing and therefore the remit of this article is to highlight specific areas of haemostatic failure, including both bleeding and thrombosis, which are relevant to ICU patients. In addition, recent advances in terms of therapeutic strategies will also be discussed.

Haemostatic reaction to vessel injury

It is important to remember in the context of this article, an overall view of the mechanisms involved in haemostasis that are illustrated schematically in Figure 3.1.

When a blood vessel becomes damaged, as a result of surgery or by a catheter, or some other means, there is some degree of local vasoconstriction. However the primary event is the adhesion of circulating platelets to the damaged vessel wall and simultaneous activation of the classical coagulation cascade, resulting in activation of thrombin and leading to the conversion of fibrinogen into fibrin. A primary haemostatic plug is produced, followed by fibrinolytic activity and hopefully repair of the damaged vessel wall. To prevent inappropriate activation of these different pathways there is now a series of very well characterised inhibitory pathways.

Platelets

Platelets were first identified as distinct corpuscles by Bizzozero in 1882, and are now known to be anucleated cell fragments derived from bone marrow. The average life span of a platelet is around ten days and about 30% are sequestered into the spleen. The normal range of the platelet count is

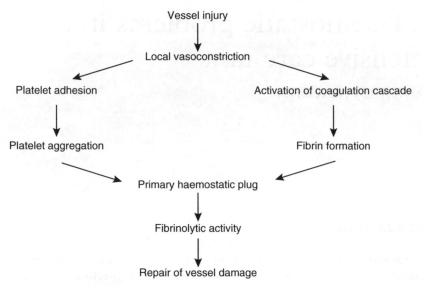

Figure 3.1 Schematic diagram of the haemostatic reaction to vessel injury.

$150–400 \times 10^9$/l, representing 5% of the total blood cell volume and 34% of the total leucocyte volume, making it the second most abundant cell.

Endothelial cell regulation of platelets

It is often forgotten that there is considerable regulation of platelet function by vascular endothelial cells. The vascular endothelial surface in the average adult is considerable, presenting a highly resistant surface to the flowing blood. The vessel wall produces several factors that affect platelet function, including prostacyclin (PGI_2), nitric oxide, and membrane-associated ATPase, which is also known as CD39. The vessel wall also expresses a thrombomodulin receptor and produces a variety of heparin and heparin-like substances, and in addition produces tissue factor pathway inhibitor (TFPI), which inhibits fibrin formation. Conversely, upon activation of the vascular endothelium, as a result of, for example sepsis, instead of producing inhibiting factors endothelial cells produce thrombotic-promoting factors, particularly tissue factor, plasmin activator inhibitor (PAI-1), Von Willebrand factor and P-selectin.

Platelet count

In Chapter 1 haemoglobin levels as triggers for transfusion were discussed, and in this chapter some triggers of platelet counting and the problems that may arise with them will be considered. Generally speaking, platelet counts above $40–50 \times 10^9/l$ are rarely associated with spontaneous bleeding although microvascular "ooze" at the traumatic lesion, surgical or otherwise, may occur. However, when platelet counts fall below $40 \times 10^9/l$, bleeding is common but not always present. We know from leukaemic patients that spontaneous bleeding does not routinely occur until the platelet count falls below $10 \times 10^9/l$, unless there is an associated platelet or coagulation disorder, which may be relevant to severely infected patients (Box 3.1).

Box 3.1 Platelet count thresholds

- Normal $150–400 \times 10^9/l$
- $>40 \times 10^9/l$ Spontaneous bleeding uncommon except
  with associated platelet dysfunction
  Bleeding only after trauma/lesion
- $<40 \times 10^9/l$ Bleeding common but not always present
- $<10 \times 10^9/l$ Severe bleeding

It is recommended that the platelet transfusion or prophylactic threshold is set at $10 \times 10^9/l$ and that is certainly the case in most leukaemia units. Obviously in critically ill patients on the ICU, there are further considerations, other traumatic bleeding for example, and individual relevant platelet transfusion thresholds may have to be pre-defined. It is important to remember however, that automated blood counters are sub-optimal in terms of precision and accuracy, particularly with platelet counts below $30 \times 10^9/l$.

When the decision to transfuse platelets has been made, some way of monitoring the benefit of transfusion is needed. There are innumerable causes of platelet refractoriness, which can be defined as a lack of response in platelet count to platelet transfusion (Box 3.2). In particular, immune refractoriness, which occurs after about eight to ten platelet transfusions, is due to the development of HLA or platelet-specific alloantibodies which bind to the transfused platelets and reduce their effectiveness. Non-immune acquired platelet refractoriness is often forgotten, and includes severe sepsis and treatment with certain antibiotic and antifungal drugs. In addition, in patients who are actively bleeding, who have disseminated intravascular coagulation (DIC) or have splenomegaly resulting in pooling in the spleen, a similar situation will exist. Transfusion of platelets may not necessarily restore platelet function (Box 3.2).

Box 3.2 Causes of refractoriness

Immune

- HLA alloantibodies
- Platelet specific antibodies
- Platelet autoantibodies
- ABO imcompatibility

Non-immune

- Sepsis
- Antibiotic/antifungal therapy
- Disseminated intravascular coagulation
- Splenomegaly

Platelet function testing

Testing of platelet function at the bedside in terms of the bleeding time is a long established screening test, but it is highly operator dependent, very poorly reproducible and it has a high false negative and false positive rate and it is poorly predictive of bleeding risk. Several other near-patient bleeding time testing devices are available (Box 3.3), reviewed by Harrison recently.[1]

Box 3.3 *In vitro* bleeding time testing devices

- Clot signature analyser
- Platelet function analyser
- Ultegra
- Thrombotic status analyser
- Thromboelastography

A thromboelastogram gives a good estimate of overall platelet function. Another relatively cheap system readily available in the United Kingdom is the platelet function analyser, in which a small volume of blood is drawn through a membrane. The device records the time to closure of the membrane and also calculates the volume of blood passing through during the closure time. This provides a very good mimic of *in vivo* primary haemostasis – in other words the ability of platelets to adhere to the hole in the membrane. This gives a very good indication of platelet transfusion requirements or indeed can also be used as a monitor of the effectiveness of transfusion.

Treatment options

Obviously the cornerstone of treatment in the patient who has bleeding associated with platelet-dysfunction or who is severely thrombocytopenic, is platelet transfusions. However, other treatment options are available which are useful in this situation (Box 3.4).

Box 3.4 Treatment options for platelet dysfunction

- Specialist care
- Vasopressin analogues
- Platelet transfusion (HLA compatible/leukodepleted)
- Tranexamic acid
- Recombinant Factor VIIa
- Bone marrow transplant

The vasopressin analogue 1-deamino-8-D-arginine vasopressin (DDAVT) has a non-specific effect on the platelet membrane and is useful in reducing platelet-type bleeding which is unresponsive to platelet transfusion. Similarly tranexamic acid, which is a fibrinolytic inhibitor, can be useful, and there are now data from several units that – if you can afford it – recombinant factor VIIa given by continuous infusion is useful in the severely bleeding thrombocytopenic platelet patient. This is presumably due to excess thrombin generation on the platelet surface, giving rise to some form of platelet clot formation.

There is also ongoing development of artificial platelets or artificial platelet membranes as putative alternatives to conventional transfusions involving allogeneic platelet concentrates, reviewed by Lee and Blajchman.[2] These include lyophilised platelets, infusible platelet membranes, red cells bearing arginine-glycine-aspartic acid ligands, fibrinogen-coated albumin microcapsules and liposome-based agents. These various products are designed to replace the use of allogeneic donor platelets with modified or artificial platelets, to augment the function of existing platelets and/or provide a pro-coagulant material capable of achieving primary haemostasis in patients with thrombocytopenia. Pre-clinical studies have been encouraging although only a few of these products have entered human trials. Safety and efficacy, however, must be demonstrated in preclinical and Phase I–III clinical trials, before these novel agents can be used clinically for patients with thrombocytopenia.

Disseminated intravascular coagulation

Box 3.5 Causes of disseminated intravascular coagulation

• Infections	Sepsis
	Viraemia
	Protozoal
• Malignancy	Metastatic carcinoma
	Leukaemia
• Obstetric	Septic abortion
	Placental abruption
	Amniotic fluid embolism
	Foetal death in utero
	Eclampsia
• Shock	Extensive trauma
	Hypovolaemic shock
	Burns
• Liver disease	
• Extracorporeal circulations	
• Intravascular haemolysis	ABO incompatibility reactions
• Transplantation rejection	
• Snake bites	

There are many possible causes of DIC seen in clinical practice, detailed in Box 3.5. About 60–70% of treatable acute DIC is caused by some form of infection process or metastatic carcinoma. Patients develop DIC as a result of inappropriate and/or excessive activation of circulating platelets and/or the coagulation cascade. Very often this is mediated by monocyte tissue factor exposure or activation of the classical contact pathway via Factor XII and Factor XI (Figure 3.2). Fibrin-platelet thrombosis occurs, which can cause end-organ damage, although very often this is not clinically apparent. What is apparent however, is that because the clotting factors and platelets have been "consumed" a low platelet count results. Generally speaking in this situation, if the platelet count falls below about $80 \times 10^9/l$, bleeding occurs. Coagulation factor deficiencies of, in particular, fibrinogen and Factor VIII

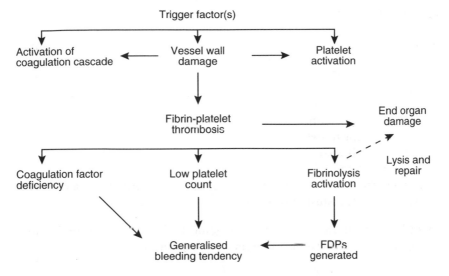

Figure 3.2 The mechanisms involved in disseminated intravascular coagulation.

along with activation of the fibrinolytic system, give rise to the classical generalised bleeding tendency of DIC. Platelet dysfunction is exacerbated by local generation of fibrinogen degradation products (Figure 3.2).

Therapy of DIC

The basic treatment of acute DIC has not really changed over the last 20 years. Early transfusion of sufficient volumes of fresh frozen plasma (12–15 ml/kg) to replace Von Willebrand factor, fibrinogen and Factor VIII are essential. Cryoprecipitate is still used in some units, also fibrinogen concentrate or platelet concentrate. Haemostatic screening tests should be monitored to try and keep the prothrombin ratio $<1\cdot5$, fibrinogen $>1\cdot0$ g/l and platelet count $>80 \times 10^9$/l.

Control of the haemorrhagic state should also be attempted. Intravascular volume should be maintained with gelatine, since dextran and starch based solutions may precipitate acquired Von Willebrand's disease. It is useful to keep the packed cell volume preferably above about 30% and certainly above 20% in the acutely bleeding situation. A certain amount of red cells improves platelet function by pushing them against the side wall of the blood vessel, reducing platelet-type intra-endothelial cell bleeding. Removal of precipitating causes such as intravenous broad-spectrum antibiotics or in the case of the obstetric patient, evacuation of the uterus, are paramount. Obviously other exacerbating factors which may make the bleeding worse, particularly hypoxia, acidosis, hypothermia, etc. should be corrected.

Heparin therapy

In my experience the benefits of heparin therapy are exceedingly limited and the risks of exacerbating the bleeding certainly outweigh any potential therapeutic benefit. There are only three definitive reasons for giving heparin – by a very low dose continuous infusion – and these are:

- patients with retention of a dead foetus where a low fibrinogen level may respond prior to delivery
- patients with disseminated neoplasm with hypofibrinogenaemia but no overt bleeding
- if you are unfortunate enough to see a patient with severe ABO haemolytic transfusion reaction.

In addition, in those patients with ongoing DIC refractive to replacement therapy, there may also be a rationale for heparin therapy.

Antithrombin

Antithrombin delays the inhibition of the classical coagulation cascade through effects on thrombin, tissue factor, and Factors IXa, Xa, XIa and XIIa. Apart from the inhibition of thrombin and other activated clotting factors, antithrombin may also down-regulate the cellular expression of pro-inflammatory cytokines.[3] Congenitally about 1 in 2000 of the population in the UK are deficient in this protein in the heterozygous form and they are at risk of developing spontaneous venothromboembolism. Naturally occurring heparans from the vascular endothelial cell specifically bind to antithrombin and accelerate by about 1000 fold its ability to bind and block the activity of thrombin. The half life of antithrombin is about 24–30 hours and the normal range in the circulation is 0·7–1·3 iu/ml. Acquired deficiency occurs during nephrotic syndrome, sepsis, DIC, liver disease and oestrogen therapy.[4-7] For example the contraceptive pill lowers antithrombin levels by about 10%.[7] Heparin therapy also lowers antithrombin by about 5% itself.

Antithrombin III (ATIII) concentrate has been available for at least the last ten years in the UK and it is potentially useful in sepsis and DIC. In a randomised trial of 35 patients with DIC due to sepsis, Fourrier et al showed that ATIII administration rapidly corrected ATIII levels and significantly reduced the duration of DIC.[4] Mortality in the ICU was non-significantly reduced in the ATIII group. Five years later, Eisele and colleagues[5] randomised 120 patients admitted to the ICU with an ATIII concentration <70% of normal to receive ATIII or placebo treatment for 5 days. Kaplan-Meier analysis showed no difference in overall survival between the two groups: 50% and 46% for ATIII and placebo, respectively. The results of ATIII treatment in this population of patients suggest that ATIII therapy reduces mortality in the sub-group of septic shock patients only. Another small trial of 42 patients with severe sepsis showed that administration of ATIII was associated with non-significant trend to a reduction in 30-day all-cause mortality and a shorter stay in the ICU.[6] A meta analysis by Levi et al. in 1999 assessed the use of antithrombin concentrate in patients with sepsis, septic shock and DIC mainly in ICU situation.[7] He showed that infusion of antithrombin concentrate to maintain levels within the normal range reduced overall mortality from 47 to 32%. A large multi-centre study of more than 2000 patients also failed to show a significant beneficial effect of ATIII on mortality in patients with sepsis.[8]

Protein C

Another advance in the treatment of DIC is offered by protein C concentrates. Protein C is another inhibitor of the classical coagulation cascade and is discussed in detail in Chapter 4. Inflammatory and coagulation processes are both affected in meningococcaemia. Severe acquired protein C deficiency in meningococcaemia is usually associated with substantial mortality: in survivors, skin grafts, amputation, and end-organ failure are not uncommon. Smith et al. assessed the effects of early replacement therapy with protein C concentrate together with continuous veno-venous haemodiafiltration and conventional treatment in 12 patients aged between 3 months and 27 years with meningococcaemia and severe acquired protein C deficiency.[9] No patients died and there were no adverse reactions to the treatment. The authors concluded that the acquired severe deficiency of protein C in meningococcaemia contributes to the pathogenesis of the thrombotic necrotic lesions in the skin and other organs and probably has an important role in the inflammatory response and suggested that a double-blind, randomised, controlled multi-centre trial was needed. A subsequent large multi-centre trial of activated protein C in adult patients with sepsis showed that recombinant human activated protein C reduced 28-day all-cause mortality, but was associated with increased incidence of bleeding of mild severity.[10] Further safety and pharmacokinetic and pharmacodynamic trials are currently being undertaken.

However, the cost of the protein C (produced by Baxter) and activated protein C (Lilly) is very high – the problem of funding the purchase of this concentrate is a major problem.

Other therapeutic options

Other therapeutic strategies are possible for the treatment of sepsis-associated acute DIC haemostatic failure.

Tissue factor pathway inhibitor (TFPI) plays a significant role in vivo in regulating coagulation resulting from exposure of blood to tissue factor after vascular injury as in the case of gram negative sepsis. In a baboon model of sepsis, highly purified recombinant TFPI was administered after *Escherichia coli* infusion.[11] Early treatment with TFPI resulted in 100% 5-day survival compared with no survivors in the placebo group and improvement of the coagulation and inflammatory responses. This compound has yet to be used in clinical trials.

Blocking the co-factor function of human tissue factor may be beneficial in various coagulation-mediated diseases. Tissue factor functions as the receptor and cofactor for Factor VIIa to form a proteolytically active tissue factor-Factor VIIa complex on cell surfaces. Monoclonal antibodies have been produced which bind to the tissue factor-Factor VIIa complex and inhibit catalytic function. These antibodies may provide a novel therapeutic option for the arrest of inappropriate triggering of coagulation by tissue factor *in vivo*.[12,13]

Anticoagulants can attenuate inflammation in animal models of sepsis with DIC and coagulation activation of human whole blood *ex vivo* results in a pro-inflammatory cytokine response.[14] This suggests that anti-inflammatory strategies such as antibodies to cytokines (for example, tumour necrosis factor α) or antagonists to cytokine receptors (for example, interleukin-1 receptor antagonist) may be another therapeutic option.

Thrombin inhibitors such as hirudin, either alone or in combination with antibiotics, have been shown to reduce mortality and improve haemostatic parameters in animal models of sepsis and DIC, but have not been used clinically.[15,16]

Aprotinin is a non-specific inhibitor of trypsin, plasmin and kallikrein. It also has some effect on platelet function. It maintains glycoprotein Ib and IIb/IIIa function on the platelet and in the patient who is bleeding, particularly after major surgery (for example, cardiac surgery) where there may well be a platelet type defect, a continuous infusion of aprotinin does seem to improve platelet function and is useful to consider in those types of situations.[17] A meta-analysis of all randomised controlled trials of the three most frequently used pharmacological strategies to decrease peri-operative blood loss during cardiac surgery (aprotinin, lysine analogues and desmopressin) was undertaken by Levi and colleagues.[17] The authors identified 72 trials (8409 patients) and concluded that pharmacological strategies which decrease peri-operative blood loss in cardiac surgery, in particular aprotinin and lysine analogues, also decrease mortality, the need for re-thoracotomy, and the proportion of patients receiving a blood transfusion.

Acquired platelet disorders

Autoimmune

The main concern to those clinicians looking after patients with acquired platelet dysfunction not related to DIC is whether this is immune type thrombocytopenia or is it associated with some drug that the patient may be receiving. Such patients do not usually bleed excessively until the platelet count falls below $5 \times 10^9/l$, since the bone marrow continues to produced very active platelets and the bleeding associated with immune or most drug type thrombocytopenias is relatively mild. Autoimmune idiopathic thrombocytopenia purpura is the most usual cause of isolated low platelet counts, is of insidious onset and is usually associated with either other autoimmune conditions or is post viral, particularly in children.

Heparin induced thrombocytopenia

Heparin induced thrombocytopenia is more of a problem. Many patients in the ICU are treated with heparin and we know that with standard unfractionated heparin the incidence of heparin induced thrombocytopenia in the UK is about 1–3%. In America it is about 15%, although the reason for the higher incidences is unclear. Even with the low molecular weight heparins the incidence of heparin induced thrombocytopenia is about 0·3%.

There are two types of heparin induced thrombocytopenia; type I is not clinically significant; the one that matters is the type II immune response to heparin. This usually manifests itself about 4 to 14 days after heparin therapy is started, and can even result from the low levels of heparin used to clean out lines. The platelet count may fall below $80 \times 10^9/l$ and about 60% of patients develop paradoxical excessive and very aggressive thrombosis, about half of which is venous and half of which is arterial. The type II condition is more likely to occur after cardiovascular surgery or peripheral vascular surgery. It has a very high morbidity and mortality if not recognised. There is some evidence in North America that if you recognise it early and treat it appropriately you can reduce this considerably. We now know the immunology of the reaction – patients produce antibodies to heparin-platelet-Factor IV complexes which then bind to a specific FCγ receptor on the platelet membrane resulting in excessive platelet activation.

Diagnosis is not simple, although an enzyme immunoassay has been developed which detects heparin-platelet-Factor IV complexes. However, the assay is very sensitive, leading to false positive results, and specificity is poor. In contrast platelet aggregation studies are insensitive but specific. Diagnosis is therefore often limited to clinical acumen.

If heparin induced thrombocytopenia is suspected, heparin therapy must be terminated and some non-heparin form of anti-thrombotic medication should be used, such as danaparoid which does not cross react with the offending antibodies. It is my view that heparin induced thrombocytopenia is still being missed as a diagnosis today and causes frequent problems. The average time to development of a fall in platelet count and the initiation of clinical thrombosis is around 8–10 days.[18]

Venous thromboembolus prophylaxis

Routine venous thromboembolus prophylaxis in the intensive care unit is another relevant issue. Patients in ICU have several problems that may preclude prophylactic heparin. They may be bleeding overtly, they may have thrombopenia or a variety of post surgical events; leg ulcer, wounds, peripheral arterial disease. There is no optimal prophylactic consensus. In a study by Hirsch and co-workers in 1995,[19] deep venous thrombosis (DVT), as detected by ultrasonography with colour Doppler imaging, was detected in 33% of 100 medical ICU patients. This unexpectedly high rate of DVT occurred despite prophylaxis in 61% and traditionally recognised risk factors failed to identify patients who developed DVT.

Two large studies in 1996 showed that subcutaneous low molecular weight heparin is as effective as unfractionated heparin for prophylaxis of thromboembolism in bedridden, hospitalised medical patients.[20,21] It therefore appears that low molecular weight heparin is the prophylactic of choice for venous thromboembolism.

Vascular access thrombosis

One area that may cause problems in ICU is vascular access thrombosis in patients with indwelling lines. The possible causes are given in Box 3.4. Hypercoagulability related to the underlying pathology is especially relevant. Increased thrombotic tendency with platelet activation and coagulation factor abnormalities that predispose to thrombosis, can be mediated through a variety of mechanisms, given in Box 3.6.

Haemofiltration

Continuous haemofiltration may be affected by premature closure or thrombosis of the filter and there are various factors that potentially contribute to this increased thrombotic tendency. The situation is compounded by loss of endothelial integrity and neutralisation of haemostatic activation. It is usually caused by aggressive activation of the contact system; Factor XIIa increases and most important of all there is increased monocyte activation via tissue factor, promoting Factor VIIa generation. This seems to be the main pathway of coagulation activation in these situations and it is compounded by again depletion of the endogenous inhibitors, particularly antithrombin and the specific heparin co-factor II. There is a marked increase of thrombin generation over the life span of the filter, and increased levels of prothrombin fragment 1 or 2 and thrombin-antithrombin complexes. Generally this is related to a reduced capacity of thrombin inhibition prior to the filtration, which increases

---

Box 3.6 Factors contributing to increased thrombotic tendency

Platelet factors

- Blood-artificial surface interaction
- Treatment with erythropoetin
- Increased platelet count
- Platelet activation

Plasma factor abnormalities

- Increased levels of Von Willebrand factor
- Hyperfibrinogenaemia
- Increased thrombin formation
- Reduced levels of protein C
- High levels of Factor VIII
- Decreased levels/activity of antithrombin III
- Impaired release of plasminogen activator
- Increased levels of antiphospholipid antibodies
- Increased levels of homocysteine

---

the blockage rate and obviously the problem. So should we replace antithrombin in this specific situation? The type of filter may matter and some types of filter are more hostile (for example, cuprophane) and some are more neutral (for example, polyacrylonitrile) than others. Perhaps lessons can be learned from cardiac pulmonary bypass, using heparin bonded circuits and supplementation of these patients with antithrombin.

Conclusion

Haemostatic failure, whether bleeding or thrombosis, is common in the ICU patient. Haematological advice can be confusing. New therapeutic options have not been adequately studied and the costs may be prohibitive.

References

1 Harrison P. Progress in the assessment of platelet function. *Br J Haematol* 2000;**111**:733–44.
2 Lee DH, Blajchman MA. Platelet substitutes and novel platelet products. *Expert Opin Investig Drugs* 2000;**9**:457–69.

3   Souter PJ, Thomas S, Hubbard AR, Poole S, Romisch J, Gray E. Antithrombin inhibits lipopolysaccharide-induced tissue factor and interleukin-6 production by mononuclear cells, human umbilical vein endothelial cells, and whole blood. *Crit Care Med* 2001;**29**:134–9.

4   Fourrier F, Chopin C, Huart JJ, Runge I, Caron C, Goudemand J. Double-blind, placebo-controlled trial of antithrombin III concentrates in septic shock with disseminated intravascular coagulation. *Chest* 1993;**104**:882–8.

5   Eisele B, Lamy M, Thijs LG, *et al.* Antithrombin III in patients with severe sepsis. A randomized, placebo-controlled, double-blind multi-center trial plus a meta-analysis on all randomized, placebo-controlled, double-blind trials with antithrombin III in severe sepsis. *Intensive Care Med* 1998;**24**:663–72.

6   Baudo F, Caimi TM, de Cataldo F, *et al.* Antithrombin III (ATIII) replacement therapy in patients with sepsis and/or postsurgical complications: a controlled double-blind, randomized, multi-center study. *Intensive Care Med* 1998;**24**:336–42.

7   Levi M, Middeldorp S, Buller HR. Oral contraceptives and hormonal replacement therapy cause an imbalance in coagulation and fibrinolysis which may explain the increased risk of venous thromboembolism. *Cardiovasc Res* 1999;**41**:21–4.

8   Fourrier F, Jourdain M, Tournoys A. Clinical trial results with antithrombin III in sepsis. *Crit Care Med* 2000;**28**:S38–S43.

9   Smith OP, White B, Vaughan D, *et al.* Use of protein-C concentrate, heparin, and haemodiafiltration in meningococcus-induced purpura fulminans. *Lancet* 1997;**350**:1590–3.

10 Bernard GR, Vincent JL, Laterre P-F, *et al.* Efficacy and safety of recombinant human activated protein C for severe sepsis. *N Engl J Med* 2001;**344**:699–709.

11 Creasey AA, Chang AC, Feigen L, Wun TC, Taylor FB Jr, Hinshaw LB. Tissue factor pathway inhibitor reduces mortality from *Escherichia coli* septic shock. *J Clin Invest* 1993;**91**:2850–6.

12 Ruf W, Edgington TS. An anti-tissue factor monoclonal antibody which inhibits TF.VIIa complex is a potent anticoagulant in plasma. *Thromb Haemost* 1991;**66**:529–33.

13 Presta L, Sims P, Meng YG, *et al.* Generation of a humanized, high affinity anti-tissue factor antibody for use as a novel antithrombotic therapeutic. *Thromb Haemost* 2001;**85**:379–89.

14 Johnson K, Choi Y, DeGroot E, Samuels I, Creasey A, Aarden L. Potential mechanisms for a proinflammatory vascular cytokine response to coagulation activation. *J Immunol* 1998;**160**:5130–5.

15 Zawilska K, Zozulinska M, Turowiecka Z, Blahut M, Drobnik L, Vinazzer H. The effect of a long-acting recombinant hirudin (PEG-hirudin) on experimental disseminated intravascular coagulation (DIC) in rabbits. *Thromb Res* 1993;**69**:315–20.

16 Dickneite G, Czech J. Combination of antibiotic treatment with the thrombin inhibitor recombinant hirudin for the therapy of experimental *Klebsiella pneumoniae* sepsis. *Thromb Haemost* 1994;**71**:768–72.

17 Levi M, Cromheecke ME, de Jonge E, *et al.* Pharmacological strategies to decrease excessive blood loss in cardiac surgery:a meta-analysis of clinically relevant endpoints. *Lancet* 1999;**354**:1940–7.

18 Boshkov LK, Warkentin TE, Hayward CP, Andrew M, Kelton JG. Heparin-induced thrombocytopenia and thrombosis. *Br J Haematol* 1993;**84**:322–8.

19 Hirsch DR, Ingenito EP, Goldhaber SZ. Prevalence of deep venous thrombosis among patients in medical intensive care. *JAMA* 1995;**274**:335–7.

20 Harenberg J, Roebruck P, Heene DL. Subcutaneous low-molecular-weight heparin versus standard heparin and the prevention of thromboembolism in

medical inpatients. The Heparin Study in Internal Medicine Group. *Haemostasis* 1996;**26**:127–39.

21 Bergmann JF, Neuhart E. A multicenter randomized double-blind study of enoxaparin compared with unfractionated heparin in the prevention of venous thromboembolic disease in elderly in-patients bedridden for an acute medical illness. The Enoxaparin in Medicine Study Group. *Thromb Haemost* 1996;**76**:529–34.

4: Activated protein C and severe sepsis

PIERRE-FRANCOIS LATERRE

Introduction

The inflammatory and pro-coagulant host responses to infection are intricately linked.[1] Infectious agents, endotoxin and inflammatory cytokines such as tumour necrosis factor alpha (TNFα) and interleukin-1 (IL-1) activate coagulation by stimulating the release of tissue factor from monocytes and endothelial cells. Upregulation of tissue factor leads to the formation of thrombin and a fibrin clot. Whilst inflammatory cytokines are capable of activating coagulation and inhibiting fibrinolysis, thrombin is capable of stimulating several inflammatory pathways.[1-5] The end result may be widespread injury to the vascular endothelium, multi-organ dysfunction, and ultimately death. Protein C is an endogenous protein – a vitamin K-dependent serine protease, which promotes fibrinolysis, whilst inhibiting thrombosis and inflammatory responses. It is therefore an important modulator of the coagulation and inflammatory pathways seen in severe sepsis.[6] Decreased protein C levels observed in patients with sepsis are associated with increased mortality. This article briefly describes the interaction between inflammation and coagulation and the role of protein C in the regulation of this interaction. The results of a large multi-centre trial of activated protein C in patients with sepsis is also presented and discussed.

Sepsis

Mortality from sepsis associated with metabolic acidosis, oliguria, hypoxaemia or shock, has remained high, even with intensive medical care, including treatment of the source of infection, intravenous fluids, nutrition, mechanical ventilation for respiratory failure, all of which are recognised standard treatments of sepsis.[7] Several treatments designed to reduce the mortality rate associated with sepsis have been unsuccessful, with the conclusion that any adjunctive therapy is destined to fail because once the clinical signs of severe sepsis are present, organ injury has already occurred.

During the initial response to infection tissue macrophages generate inflammatory cytokines, including TNFα, IL-1, and IL-8[8] in response to bacterial cell wall products. Although cytokines play an important part in host defence by attracting activated neutrophils to the site of infection, inappropriate and excessive release into the systemic circulation may lead to widespread microvascular injury and multi-organ failure.[9] Most of the previous clinical trials have evaluated agents designed to attenuate these early inflammatory events in sepsis, including glucocorticoids and antagonists to endotoxin, TNFα and IL-1.[10] None of these treatments have been effective, perhaps in part because the importance of the coagulation cascade in sepsis was not recognised.

Several pro-coagulant mechanisms have been associated with decreased survival in critically ill patients with sepsis. Non-survivors have been found to have elevated levels of plasminogen activator inhibitor type-1 (PAI-1), an inhibitor of normal fibrinolysis, and decreased levels of antithrombin III and protein C.[11] There are important molecular links between the pro-coagulant and inflammatory mechanisms in the pathogenesis of organ failure in patients with sepsis.[12]

The interaction of inflammation and coagulation

The activation of the coagulation pathway, especially in severe sepsis, appears to be mediated initially by tissue factor expression in response to endotoxin and other mediators, resulting in conversion of pro-thrombin to thrombin via factor X-Va complexes. Although thrombin is usually considered a pro-coagulant, it also has relevant homeostatic anti-coagulant effects. Thrombomodulin on the surface of endothelial cells binds thrombin, thus blocking thrombin-mediated fibrinogen, platelet and factor V pro-coagulant activity. Instead, the thrombin–thrombomodulin complex activates protein C via another site on the thrombin molecule, and results in initiation of the activated protein C pathway. Specific receptors called the endothelial cell protein C receptors – or EPCR, mediate this process. Activated protein C then dissociates from the EPCR, binds to its non-enzymatic co-factor, protein S, and, through inactivation of factor Va, exerts anti-coagulant activity.

Protein C and the microvasculature

Protein C is particularly important in the microcirculation, which is especially relevant in sepsis. Although the number of thrombomodulin molecules per endothelial cell is approximately constant, the local concentration of thrombomodulin is determined by the number of endothelial cells that are in contact with the blood. Since the endothelial cell surface area per unit of blood volume is much greater within the microcirculation than in larger blood vessels, the concentration of thrombomodulin is also higher. This means that thrombin is rapidly removed from the microcirculation by binding to thrombomodulin. The activated protein C system has a particular role in the regulation of coagulopathies in the microcirculation, confirmed in clinical studies.[13]

Thrombin

Thrombin is also involved in the process of inflammation, by activating P-selectin expression on endothelial cells, resulting in neutrophil and monocyte adhesion. Thrombin is chemotactic for polymorphonuclear leucocytes and induces platelet-activating factor (PAF) formation by endothelial cells, which is a potent activator of neutrophils. In addition, thrombin is capable of stimulating multiple inflammatory pathways and further suppressing the endogenous fibrinolytic system by activating thrombin-activatable fibrinolysis inhibitor (TAFI).

Activity of $\alpha_1$antitrypsin is increased as part of the acute phase response, inhibiting the protein C pathway. Cytokines such as TNFα and endotoxin amplify tissue factor expression by monocytes, triggering further coagulation. Concurrent complement activation by endotoxin also propagates the coagulation response and levels of both fibrinogen. PAI-1 is a potent inhibitor of tissue plasminogen activator, the endogenous pathway for lysing a fibrin clot, and which may also be increased as part of the inflammatory response. Cytokines and thrombin can both impair the endogenous fibrinolytic potential by stimulating the release of PAI-1 from platelets and endothelial cells.

Protein C activity

Clearly an endogenous mechanism to disrupt the amplification of coagulation during inflammation is essential to prevent detrimental widespread effects. Endogenous activated protein C modulates both coagulation and inflammatory responses and thus interferes with the inflammation-mediated exacerbation of coagulation. Activated protein C can intervene at multiple points during the systemic response to infection. It exerts an anti-thrombotic effect by inactivating factors Va and VIIIa, limiting the generation of thrombin. As a result of decreased thrombin levels, the thrombin-mediated inflammatory, pro-coagulant, and anti-fibrinolytic response is attenuated. *In vitro* data indicate that activated protein C exerts an anti-inflammatory effect by inhibiting the production of TNFα, IL-1, and IL-6 by monocytes and limiting monocyte and neutrophil adhesion to the endothelium.[14] Activated protein C promotes fibrinolysis by forming a tight complex with PAI-1; once the complex with activated protein C forms, PIA-1 can no longer inhibit tissue plasminogen activator. Because of the ability of the activated protein C to limit thrombin generation, it can also reduce the activation of TAFI which functions by removing lysine residues from the fibrin clot, which would normally stimulate plasminogen activation and the fibrinolytic activity of plasmin.

Protein C in sepsis

The conversion of protein C to activated protein C may be impaired during sepsis.[15] There are several reasons why activated protein C might be an effective therapy in patients with sepsis. Firstly, most patients with severe sepsis have diminished levels of activated protein C, in part because the inflammatory cytokines generated in sepsis downregulate thrombomodulin and ECPR, which are essential for the conversion of inactive protein C to activated protein C.[16] Secondly, activated protein C inhibits activated factors V and VIII, thereby decreasing the formation of thrombin.[16] Thirdly, activated protein C stimulates fibrinolysis by reducing the concentration of PAI-1. Also, studies in baboons demonstrated that exogenous protein C administration decreased mortality and the coagulopathies associated with infusion of lethal concentration of *Escherichia coli*.[17] Conversely, antibodies against protein C increased mortality. Reduced levels of protein C are found in the majority of patients with sepsis and are associated with an increased risk of death.[18-21] In addition treatment with protein C has been suggested to improve clinical outcomes in patients with severe meningococcaemia[22] and protein C measurement may provide a prognostic marker for hypercoagulable states and thus unfavourable outcome.[23]

Previous pre-clinical and clinical studies showed that the administration of activated protein C may improve the outcome of severe sepsis. In a placebo-controlled phase 2 trial in patients with severe sepsis, an infusion of recombinant human activated protein C (Eli Lilly, Indianapolis), resulted in dose-dependent reductions in the plasma levels of D-dimer and serum levels of IL-6 as markers of coagulopathy and inflammation respectively.[24]

A multi-centre trial was therefore undertaken to evaluate mortality benefit and safety profile of administration of human recombinant activated protein C in patients with severe sepsis.[25] Activated protein C was produced from an established mammalian cell line into which the complementary DNA for human protein C had been inserted.[26] Eligible patients were enrolled into a randomised, double-blind, placebo-controlled trial, conducted at 164 centres in 11 countries from July 1998 until June 2000. The criteria for severe sepsis were a modification of those defined by Bone *et al.*[27] Patients were eligible for the trial if they had a known or suspected infection on the basis of clinical data at the time of screening and if they met the following criteria within a 24-hour period: three or more signs of systemic inflammation and sepsis-induced dysfunction of at least one organ or system that lasted no longer than 24 hours. Patients had to begin treatment within 24 hours after meeting the inclusion criteria. Patients were randomly assigned through a centralised randomisation centre to receive either activated protein C (*drotrecogin alfa activated*) or placebo. Block randomisation, stratified according to the investigating site, was used. Activated protein C (24 micrograms/kg/h) or placebo was administered intravenously at a constant rate for a total of 96 hours. The infusion was interrupted 1 hour before any percutaneous procedure or major surgery and was resumed 1 hour and 12 hours later, respectively, in the absence of bleeding complications. Clinicians continued with their management strategies according to usual practice.

Evaluation of patients

Patients were followed for 28 days after infusion or until death. Baseline characteristics including demographic information and information on pre-existing conditions, organ function, markers of disease severity, infection, and haematological and other laboratory tests were assessed within 24 hours before the infusion was begun. D-dimer levels and IL-6 were measured at baseline, and on days 1–7, 14 and 28 were assayed using commercially available latex agglutination test and enzyme immunoassay kits, respectively. Neutralising antibodies against activated protein C were also measured. Microbiological cultures were assessed at baseline and when indicated until day 28. Patients were defined as having a deficiency of protein C if their plasma protein C activity level was below the lower limit of normal (81%) within 24 hours before the initiation of infusion, but this information was not made available to the investigators – these data were predefined for post-study analysis.

The primary efficacy end point was death from any cause and was assessed 28 days after the initiation of the infusion. The prospectively defined primary analysis included all patients who received the infusion for any length of time, with patients analysed according to the treatment group to which they were assigned at randomisation. The trial was designed to enrol 2280 patients; two planned interim analyses by an independent data and safety monitoring board took place after 760 and 1520 patients had been enrolled. Statistical guidelines to suspend enrolment if activated protein C was found to be significantly more efficacious than placebo were determined *a priori*.

Results

Enrolment was suspended following the second interim analysis of data from 1520 patients because the differences in the mortality rate between the two groups was greater than the *a priori* guideline for stopping the trial. Therefore the results presented here include data from these 1520 patients plus additional patients who were enrolled before the completion of the second interim analysis (total = 1728).

Baseline patient characteristics

Of 1728 patients who underwent randomisation, 1690 actually received the study drug or placebo. At baseline, the demographic characteristics and severity of disease were similar in patients in the placebo group and the activated protein C group. Approximately 75% of the patients had at least two dysfunctional organs or systems at the time of enrolment. The incidence of gram-positive and gram-negative infections was similar within each group and between the two groups. Baseline levels of indicators of coagulopathy and inflammation were also similar in the two groups. Protein C deficiency was present in 87·6% of the patients in whom results were available.

Efficacy

Twenty-eight days after the start of the infusion, 30·8% of patients in the placebo group and 24·7% of patients in the activated protein C group had died. This difference in the all cause mortality was significant (P = 0·005 in the non-stratified analysis) and was associated with an absolute reduction in the risk of death of 6·1%. The prospectively defined primary analysis in which the groups were stratified according to the baseline APACHE II score, age, and protein C activity produced similar results (P = 0·005), as did the analysis including the 38 patients who underwent randomisation but who never received the infusion (P = 0·003). The results of the prospectively defined primary analysis represent a reduction in the relative risk of death of 19·4% (95% confidence interval 6·6–30·5%) in association with treatment with activated protein C, compared with placebo. A Kaplan-Meier analysis of survival yielded similar results (P = 0·006) (Figure 4.1). The absolute difference in survival between the two groups was evident within days after the initiation of the infusion and continued to increase throughout the remainder of the study period.

Prospectively defined subgroup analyses were performed for a number of baseline characteristics, including APACHE II score, organ dysfunction, other indicators of the severity of disease, sex, age, the site of infection, the type of infection (gram-positive, gram-negative, or mixed), and presence or absence of protein C deficiency. A consistent effect of treatment with activated protein C was observed in all the subgroups including those patients both with protein C deficiency and those with normal protein C levels.

D-Dimer and interleukin-6 concentrations

Plasma D-dimer levels were significantly lower in those patients in the activated protein C group than in patients in the placebo group, during the infusion period (Figure 4.2). Activated protein C was also associated with

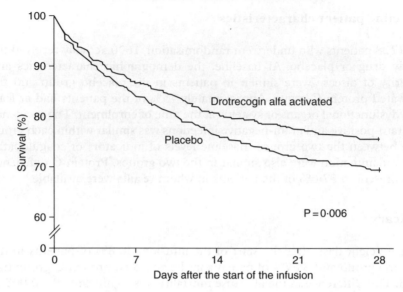

Figure 4.1 Kaplan-Meier estimates of survival in patients with severe sepsis in the activated protein C (Drotrecogin alfa activated) group (n = 850) and patients with severe sepsis in the placebo group (n = 840). Reproduced with permission from Bernard G, et al. N Engl J Med 2001;344:699–709.[24]

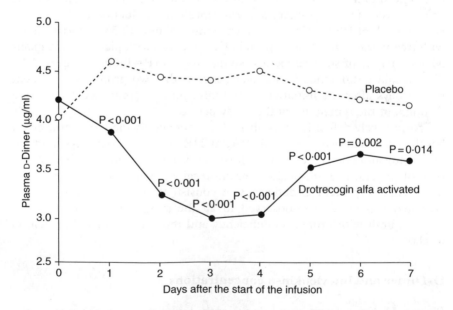

Figure 4.2 Median plasma D-dimer levels in patients with severe sepsis in the activated protein C (Drotrecogin alfa activated) group (n = 770) and patients with severe sepsis in the placebo group (n = 729). Reproduced with permission from Bernard G, et al. N Engl J Med 2001;344:699–709.[24]

greater attenuation of the increase in serum IL-6 concentrations than in the patients in the placebo group on day 1 and on days 4, 5, 6, and 7.

Complications

The percentage of patients who had at least one serious adverse event was similar in both patient groups. The incidence of serious bleeding was higher, however, in the activated protein C group than in the placebo group (3·5% vs. 2·0%, P = 0·06). This difference in the incidence of serious bleeding was observed only during the infusion period; after this time, the incidence was similar in the two groups. Among the patients who received activated protein C, the incidence of serious bleeding was similar for those who received activated protein C alone and in those who also received heparin. In both the activated protein C group and the placebo group, serious bleeding occurred mainly in those patients with some predisposition to bleeding, such as gastrointestinal ulceration, an activated partial-thromboplastin time (aPTT) of more than 120 seconds, a prolonged prothrombin time (PT), a platelet count which fell below 30 000/ml and remained at that level despite standard therapy, traumatic injury of a blood vessel, or traumatic injury of a highly vascular organ. There was a fatal intracranial haemorrhage in two patients in the activated protein C group during the infusion (one on day 1 and one on day 4) and in one patient in the placebo group six days after the end of the infusion. After adjustment for the duration of survival, blood transfusion requirements were similar in both groups.

There were no other safety concerns associated with treatment with activated protein C on the basis of assessments of organ dysfunction, vital signs, biochemical data, or haematological data. The incidence of thrombotic events was similar in the two groups. The incidence of new infections was around 25% in both groups of patients, and neutralising antibodies to activated protein C were not detected in any patient.

Discussion

In this study, the administration of activated protein C reduced the rate of death from any cause at 28 days in patients with a clinical diagnosis of severe sepsis, resulting in a 19·4% reduction in the relative risk of death and an absolute reduction of 6·1%.[24] A survival benefit was evident throughout the 28-day study period, whether or not the groups were stratified according to the severity of disease. These results indicate that in this population, 1 additional life would be saved for every 16 patients treated with activated protein C.

In patients with severe sepsis, the benefit of activated protein C is most likely explained by its biological activity. Activated protein C inhibits the generation of thrombin through inactivation of factor Va and factor VIIIa.[28,29] A reduction in the generation of thrombin was seen as greater decreases in plasma D-dimer levels during the first seven days after the infusion was initiated in patients treated with activated protein C compared with the patients who received placebo. The rise in D-dimer levels after the end of the 96-hour infusion of activated protein C suggests that longer periods of infusion of activated protein C may be associated with a greater benefit in terms of survival.

Treatment with activated protein C decreased inflammation, as shown by decreases in IL-6 levels, as might be expected given the anti-inflammatory activity of activated protein C. Such activity may be mediated indirectly through the inhibition of thrombin generation, which leads to decreased activation of platelets, recruitment of neutrophils, and degranulation of mast cells.[2] Furthermore, pre-clinical studies have shown that activated protein C has direct anti-inflammatory properties, including inhibition of neutrophil activation, decreased monocyte cytokine release, and inhibition of E-selectin–mediated adhesion of cells to vascular endothelium.[30–32]

The effect of treatment with activated protein C was consistent whether or not patients were stratified according to age, APACHE II score, sex, number of dysfunctional organs or systems, site or type of infection, or the presence or absence of protein C deficiency at study entry. Since reductions in the relative risk of death were observed regardless of whether patients had protein C deficiency at baseline, it is suggested that activated protein C has pharmacological effects beyond merely replacement of depleted endogenous levels. This observation suggests that measurements of protein C are not necessary to identify which patients would benefit from treatment with the drug.

Bleeding was the most common adverse event associated with activated protein C administration, consistent with its known anti-thrombotic activity. The incidence of serious bleeding suggests that 1 additional serious bleeding event would occur for every 66 patients treated with activated protein C. Serious bleeding tended to occur in patients with pre-disposing conditions, such as gastrointestinal ulceration, traumatic injury of a blood vessel or highly vascular organ injury, or markedly abnormal coagulation parameters (for example, platelet count, aPTT, PT). The incidence of thrombotic events was not increased by treatment with activated protein C, and the anti-inflammatory effect was not associated with an increased incidence of new infections.

In summary, the biological activity of activated protein C was demonstrated by the finding of greater decreases in D-dimer and IL-6 levels in patients who received the drug than in those who received placebo. The higher incidence of serious bleeding during infusion in the activated protein C group is consistent with the anti-thrombotic activity of the drug and occurred mainly in patients with increased bleeding risk. In patients with severe sepsis, an intravenous infusion of activated protein C at a dose of 24 micrograms/kg/h for 96 hours was associated with a significant reduction in mortality and an acceptable safety profile. Nevertheless, it should be noted that the study excluded patients with a higher risk of bleeding, such as those with chronic liver disease, chronic renal failure who were dependent on dialysis, organ transplant recipients, patients with thrombocytopenia, and those who had taken aspirin in the three days before the study. Many patients with severe sepsis meet one or more of these criteria. Also, patients less than 18 years of age were excluded from the trial. Further studies to assess the safety of activated protein C are now underway, and include paediatric use.

References

1   Esmon CT, Taylor FB Jr, Snow TR. Inflammation and coagulation: linked processes potentially regulated through a common pathway mediated by protein C. *Thromb Haemost* 1991;**66**:160–5.

2   Yan SB, Grinnell BW. Recombinant human protein C, protein S, and thrombomomodulin as anti-thrombotics. *Perspect Drug Discovery Des* 1993; **1**:503–20.

3   Stouthard JM, Levi M, Hack CE, *et al.* Interleukin-6 stimulates coagulation, not fibrinolysis, in humans. *Thromb Haemost* 1996;**76**:738–42.

4   Conkling PR, Greenberg CS, Weinberg JB. Tumor necrosis factor induces tissue factor-like activity in human leukemia cell line U937 and peripheral blood monocytes. *Blood* 1988;**72**:128–33.

5   Bevilacqua MP, Pober JS, Majeau GR, Fiers W, Cotran RS, Gimbrone MA Jr. Recombinant tumor necrosis induces procoagulant activity in cultured human vascular endothelium: characterization and comparison with the actions of interleukin 1. *Proc Natl Acad Sci USA* 1986;**12**:4533–7.

6   Esmon CT. The protein C anticoagulant pathway. *Arterioscler Thromb* 1992;**12**:135–45.

7   Rangel-Frausto MS, Pittet D, Costigan M, Hwang T, Davis CS, Wenzel RS. The natural history of the systemic inflammatory response syndrome (SIRS): a prospective study. *JAMA* 1995;**273**:117–23.

8   Parrillo JE. Pathogenetic mechanisms of septic shock. *N Engl J Med* 1993;**328**:1471–7.

9   Kurahashi K, Kajikawa O, Sawa T, *et al.* Pathogenesis of septic shock in *Pseudomonas aeruginosa* pneumonia. *J Clin Invest* 1999;**104**:743–50.

10 Wheeler AP, Bernard GR. Treating patients with severe sepsis. *N Engl J Med* 1999;**340**:207–14.

11 Lorente JA, Garcia-Frade LJ, Landin L, *et al.* Time course of hemostatic abnormalities in sepsis and its relation to outcome. *Chest* 1993;**103**:1536–42.

12 Esmon CT. Introduction: are natural anticoagulants candidates for modulating the inflammatory response to endotoxin? *Blood* 2000;**95**:1113–16.

13 Fuentes-Prior P, Iwanaga Y, Huber R, *et al.* Structural basis for the anticoagulant activity of the thrombin–thrombomodulin complex. *Nature* 2000;**404**:518–24.

14 White B, Schmidt M, Murphy C, *et al.* Activated protein C inhibits lipopolysaccharide-induced nuclear translocation of nuclear factor kappaB (NF-kappaB) and tumour necrosis factor alpha (TNF alpha) production in the THP-1 monocytic cell line. *Br J Haematol* 2000;**110**:130–4.

15 Boehme MW, Deng Y, Raeth U, *et al.* Release of thrombomodulin from endothelial cells by concerted action of TNF-alpha and neutrophils: *in vivo* and *in vitro* studies. *Immunology* 1996;**87**:134–40.

16 Esmon CT. Regulation of blood coagulation. *Biochim Biophys Acta* 2000;**1477**:349–60.

17 Taylor FB Jr, Chang A, Esmon CT, D'Angelo A, Vigano-D'Angelo S, Blick KE. Protein C prevents the coagulopathic and lethal effects of *Escherichia coli* infusion in the baboon. *J Clin Invest* 1987;**79**:918–25.

18 Fourrier F, Chopin C, Goudemand J, *et al.* Septic shock, multiple organ failure, and disseminated intravascular coagulation: compared patterns of antithrombin III, protein C, and protein S deficiencies. *Chest* 1992;**101**:816–23.

19 Lorente JA, Garcia-Frade LJ, Landin L, *et al.* Time course of hemostatic abnormalities in sepsis and its relation to outcome. *Chest* 1993;**103**:1536–42.

20 Boldt J, Papsdorf M, Rothe A, Kumle B, Piper S. Changes of the hemostatic network in critically ill patients – is there a difference between sepsis, trauma, and neurosurgery patients? *Crit Care Med* 2000;**28**:445–50.

21 Powars D, Larsen R, Johnson J, *et al.* Epidemic meningococcemia and purpura fulminans with induced protein C deficiency. *Clin Infect Dis* 1993;**17**:254–61.

22 White B, Livingstone W, Murphy C, Hodgson A, Rafferty M, Smith OP. An open-label study of the role of adjuvant hemostatic support with protein C replacement therapy in purpura fulminans-associated meningococcemia. *Blood* 2000;**96**:3719–24.

23 Mesters RM, Helterbrand J, Utterback BG, *et al.* Prognostic value of protein C concentrations in neutropenic patients at high risk of severe septic complications. *Crit Care Med* 2000;**28**:2209–16.

24 Hartman DL, Bernard GR, Helterbrand JD, Yan SB, Fisher CJ. Recombinant human activated protein C (rhAPC) improves coagulation abnormalities associated with severe sepsis. *Intensive Care Med* 1998;**24**(Suppl 1):S77 (abstract).

25 Bernard GR, Vincent J-L, Laterre P-F, *et al.* for The Recombinant Human Activated Protein C Worldwide Evaluation in Severe Sepsis (PROWESS) Study Group. Efficacy and Safety of Recombinant Human Activated Protein C for Severe Sepsis. *N Engl J Med* 2001;**344**:699–709.

26 Yan SC, Razzano P, Chao YB, *et al.* Characterization and novel purification of recombinant human protein C from three mammalian cell lines. *Biotechnology* 1990;**8**:655–61.

27 Bone RC, Balk RA, Cerra FB, *et al.* Definitions for sepsis and organ failure and guidelines for the use of innovative therapies in sepsis. *Chest* 1992;**101**:1644–55.

28 Walker FJ, Sexton PW, Esmon CT. The inhibition of blood coagulation by activated protein C through the selective inactivation of activated factor V. *Biochim Biophys Acta* 1979;**571**:333–42.

29 Fulcher CA, Gardiner JE, Griffin JH, Zimmerman TS. Proteolytic inactivation of human factor VIII procoagulant protein by activated human protein C and its analogy with factor V. *Blood* 1984;**63**:486–9.

30 Grey ST, Tsuchida A, Hau H, Orthner CL, Salem HH, Hancock WW. Selective inhibitory effects of the anticoagulant activated protein C on the responses of human mononuclear phagocytes to LPS, IFN-gamma, or phorbol ester. *J Immunol* 1994;**153**:3664–72 (abstract).

31 Hirose K, Okajima K, Taoka Y, *et al.* Activated protein C reduces the ischemia/reperfusion-induced spinal cord injury in rats by inhibiting neutrophil activation. *Ann Surg* 2000;**232**:272–80.

32 Grinnell BW, Hermann RB, Yan SB. Human protein C inhibits selectin-mediated cell adhesion: role of unique fucosylated oligosaccharide. *Glycobiology* 1994;**4**:221–5.

5: Transfusion-related acute lung injury

ANDREW BODENHAM, SHEILA MacLENNAN,
SIMON V BAUDOUIN

Introduction

Transfusion related lung injury has been reported to occur in about 0·2% of all transfused patients, although it is thought that this may be an underestimate. The lung injury may be severe enough to warrant admission to the intensive care unit for ventilation, and is similar to acute respiratory distress syndrome in many respects. The exact cause of lung injury after transfusion remains confusing, although it is suggested to be due to the presence of donor antibodies. This article describes the clinical manifestations, possible causes and similarity to other lung conditions of transfusion related lung injury and suggests future research strategies.

What is transfusion-related lung injury?

Transfusion-related acute lung injury (TRALI) is a rare and poorly defined syndrome of acute respiratory failure of non-cardiac origin. It is clinically indistinguishable from acute respiratory distress syndrome (ARDS), or its less severe form, acute lung injury (ALI), and usually occurs within four hours of a transfusion episode, although it may occur up to 24 hours after transfusion.[1] TRALI is thought to be caused by the interaction of leucocyte antibodies (usually donor-derived) and leucocyte antigens. Although rare, it is a significant cause of transfusion-associated morbidity and mortality and has been reported as the third most common cause of fatal transfusion reactions. Although blood transfusion is often cited as being a cause of ARDS, TRALI may in fact be a distinct entity. The prognosis differs from ARDS arising from other causes and patients may only have single organ failure – the lungs. If the patient survives the acute event there are usually no long-term sequelae.

Clinical manifestations

TRALI is characterised clinically by symptoms and signs of dyspnoea, cyanosis, hypotension, fever and chills and pulmonary oedema. The symptoms typically begin within one to two hours of transfusion and are usually present by four to six hours, with the severity ranging from mild to severe. A significant proportion of reported patients have sufficiently severe lung dysfunction to require mechanical ventilation. However, it is only the more severe cases that are likely to be reported to local transfusion centres. For this reason it is unclear whether the disorder may also occur in a much milder form, which may not be reported.

TRALI is most often associated with the transfusion of whole blood, packed red blood cells (pRBCs) or fresh frozen plasma (FFP), although there are rare reports of TRALI following transfusion of granulocytes, cryoprecipitate, platelet concentrates and apheresis platelets. Infusion of even very small volumes of blood products can trigger lung injury.

TRALI is essentially a clinical diagnosis in the first instance, as laboratory confirmation of the condition is not possible for some weeks. In addition some apparently clear-cut cases may have had no positive laboratory confirmation.

What causes TRALI?

TRALI is considered to be the result of the interaction of (usually) donor-derived specific leucocyte antibodies with patient-derived leucocytes. However, in some cases reported to SHOT (Serious Hazard of Transfusion),[2,3] no donor antibodies have been identified despite extensive investigation, although of course, it is possible that these cases were misdiagnosed. Conversely, it is known that not all transfusions of components containing anti-leucocyte antibodies result in TRALI. In a recent retrospective study it was evident that almost all donors studied who have been implicated in TRALI reactions have previously donated on many occasions without the transfusion resulting in TRALI. In addition other components produced from the same donation have been transfused without similar sequelae. Nearly half of the 44 cases of TRALI reported to SHOT had either pre-existing cardiac or pulmonary disease, but it is not clear whether this is because this population is more heavily transfused or because such disease predisposes to the development of TRALI.

It has been postulated that, in addition to the transfusion of anti-leucocyte antibodies, a second "hit" is required for the development of the syndrome. Hypoxia, recent surgery, cytokine therapy, active infection or inflammation, massive transfusion, and biologically active lipids present in stored (but not fresh) cellular components have all been implicated.[4,5] The transfusion of leucocyte antibodies itself may act as a "second hit" in a patient whose leucocytes are already activated by other risk factors such as cardiopulmonary bypass or sepsis.

Incidence of TRALI

The best estimates of the incidence of TRALI come from institutions which have a high interest in the syndrome: Popovsky and Moore[1] quote a rate of 0·02% of all transfused blood components, or 0·16% of all patients transfused. TRALI may occur elsewhere but be unrecognised, and therefore overall incidence may be underestimated; this is supported by the UK Serious Hazards of Transfusion reporting system (SHOT) data, in which an average of 15 cases occurred each year over 3 years from approximately 2·5 million donations per annum (Figure 5.1).[2,3]

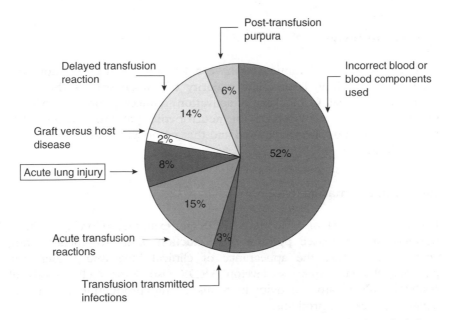

Figure 5.1 In November 1996 haematologists in the United Kingdom and Ireland were invited on a voluntary confidential basis to inform Serious Hazards of Transfusion (SHOT) of deaths and major adverse events in seven categories associated with the transfusion of red cells, platelets, fresh frozen plasma, or cryoprecipitate. This pie chart gives an overview of 366 cases for which initial report forms were received. There was at least one death in every category. Reproduced with permission from Williamson LM, et al. BMJ 1999;319:16–19.[3]

ARDS and TRALI

The relationship between the ARDS and TRALI remains controversial. The clinical, radiological and haemodynamic findings in the two syndromes are identical,[5-7] although survival following TRALI seems significantly better than in ARDS where mortality of at least 40% is reported.[8] Mortality in ARDS is related to the severity of the precipitating illness rather than to the degree of pulmonary dysfunction and this may explain the apparent differences in outcome. It is therefore likely that TRALI and ARDS share common mechanisms and an understanding of the pathophysiology of ARDS will contribute to that of TRALI. The pathophysiology of ARDS, as shown by post-mortem studies, is one of diffuse damage to alveolar units.[9] Both epithelial and endothelial injury occur and the alveolar spaces are filled with fluid and proteinaceous debris. Histological studies show an intense acute inflammatory cell infiltrate of both neutrophils and monocytes, migrating across the pulmonary vascular bed into the alveolar spaces. The inflammatory nature of ARDS has been intensively investigated in the last decade and a number of conclusions have been drawn.[9–11]

Role of leucocytes

Both neutrophils and monocytes have a key role in the initiation and perpetuation of lung injury. The majority of animal studies show that neutrophil removal, or blockage of activation, reduces or prevents ARDS. Occasional reports of ARDS in neutropenic patients suggest that neutrophils are not always required and that monocytes alone may initiate the syndrome.

Role of inflammation

Patients at high risk of developing ARDS (for example, following multiple trauma) have increased pulmonary production of neutrophil attracting chemokines, before the appearance of clinical lung injury. High-risk patients who subsequently develop ARDS also show higher levels of systemic inflammatory activity in terms of the production of reactive oxygen species and products.

Role of interleukin-8 and severity of ARDS

Broncho-alveolar lavage studies of patients and animals show intense inflammatory activity within the alveolar spaces in lung injury, both in terms of cells and mediators. Persistent inflammatory activity is also a mark of poorer outcome in ARDS. It has been shown that levels of tumour necrosis factor and interleukin-8 (IL-8) in the bronchoalveolar lavage fluid correlate with the severity of ARDS.[12]

It is possible to produce a paradigm for the initiation of acute lung injury based on the research performed in the last decade. In this paradigm, systemic inflammatory stimuli in terms of both cellular and circulating mediators, released during a number of severe illnesses, activate and damage the pulmonary endothelial/epithelial interface. Local production of further pro-inflammatory mediators occurs with further recruitment of inflammatory cells. This inflammatory damage results in increased vascular permeability causing the observed fall in gas exchange and development of acute pulmonary oedema.

TRALI and the acute inflammatory response

There is substantial evidence that the acute inflammatory response also plays a central role in TRALI.[5-7] A number of reports suggest that systemic leucocyte activation, complement consumption and the release of pro-inflammatory cytokines occur during TRALI. In one well-documented example a healthy volunteer developed TRALI after receiving an experimental intravenous gammaglobulin concentrate containing a high titre of monocyte-reactive IgG antibody.[13] Serial blood samples taken during the study showed a significant fall in the number of circulating neutrophils and monocytes, increases in circulating tumour necrosis factor α (TNFα), IL-6 and IL-8, complement activation and consumption, and the release of soluble neutrophil degranulation products. The volunteer required a period of mechanical ventilation but ultimately made a full recovery.

Further evidence for a central role for inflammation in TRALI comes from a case report of a 58-year-old man who died following the acute onset of pulmonary oedema following a platelet transfusion.[14] Post-mortem findings were indistinguishable from those seen in classic early ARDS with granulocyte aggregation in the pulmonary microvasculature. Electron microscopy revealed capillary endothelial damage with activated granulocytes in contact with the alveolar basement membrane.

The pro-inflammatory initiating event in the majority of cases of TRALI is likely to be the transfusion of donor-acquired complement and leucocyte activating antibodies. In one series of 36 cases, 89% of patients had evidence of the passive transfer of leukoagglutinin-type antibodies.[1] However, these cannot always be detected in many cases of TRALI, and conversely, many patients who receive transfusions containing these antibodies, which are estimated to be present in 7·7% of multiparous blood donations,[15] do not develop lung injury.

Does TRALI contribute to ARDS?

ARDS is a final common pathway following a range of non-pulmonary insults and although several clinical conditions are associated with the development of ARDS, relatively few studies have attempted to assess the risk of developing ARDS following a given insult.[16] Such studies are also limited by the inclusion of only those patients already within intensive care units (usually North American). However, these studies do indicate that a number of conditions carry a high risk of developing ARDS, including septic shock, necrotising pancreatitis, severe multiple trauma and cardio-pulmonary bypass surgery. Massive blood transfusion, which was variably defined in the studies, is also associated with an increased risk of acute lung injury. Many patients had multiple risk factors present and therefore it is not possible to assess the contribution that each of these factors, and possibly other as yet unknown factors, makes to the development of ARDS. It is possible that some of the cases of ARDS are related in whole or in part to TRALI. This may be one explanation for the association of ARDS and blood transfusion. A "double hit" mechanism may also be relevant, as most cases of ARDS have multiple risk factors present.

Laboratory investigations

The objective of laboratory investigations of patients with suspected TRALI is to confirm the presence of a leucocyte antibody, which would support the clinical diagnosis of TRALI. In UK laboratories, investigations for TRALI are performed within the National Blood Service. The hospital blood bank should be informed as soon as the diagnosis is suspected, so that the appropriate Regional Blood Centre can be informed. This is necessary as several components may have been made from one donor unit and these components should be put on hold or recalled if not already transfused, whilst the investigation is under way.

Clotted and blood samples anticoagulated with EDTA should be obtained from the patient, initially for the detection of leucocyte antibodies, and later to perform leucocyte and/or granulocyte antigen typing if antibodies have been found in the donor unit. Sometimes a strong antibody in donor plasma can be picked up in the recipient serum soon after transfusion, but this passive antibody is then no longer present when a second sample is tested a month later. The Transfusion Centre will also investigate samples from the donor(s) for the presence of leucocyte or granulocyte antibodies. These antibodies are most often present in multiparous female donors, but are also sometimes found in the serum of donors who have themselves been previously transfused.

If antibodies are found in donor serum, then the patient sample will be investigated for the corresponding leucocyte or granulocyte antigen. Conversely if antibodies are found in the recipient's serum then donor samples will be investigated in this way. An alternative method of assessing a possible leucocyte antigen antibody interaction is to perform a cross-match of the donor serum against recipient's white cells. A fresh sample from the patient is required for this.

Treatment options

There is no specific treatment for TRALI. As with ARDS/ALI from other causes the precipitating cause should be removed as soon as it is recognised. Thereafter treatment is largely supportive, to allow time for lung injury to resolve. Steroids have been advocated in this condition but proof of efficacy is lacking.

Future research directions

The incidence of TRALI and its importance as a cause of ARDS/ALI needs to be determined by further studies. The role of donor antibodies, the age of blood products and biologically active lipids and also patient factors, in the aetiology of TRALI are poorly understood. Better understanding of the disease would enable blood transfusion services to make more informed decisions in an attempt to reduce morbidity and mortality associated with TRALI, for example, avoiding the use of products containing multiple antibodies for critically ill patients already at risk of lung injury.

References

1 Popovsky MA, Moore SB. Diagnostic and pathogenetic considerations in transfusion-related acute lung injury. *Transfusion* 1985;**25**:573–7.
2 Serious Hazards of Transfusion (SHOT). Annual Reports 1996–7, 1997–8, 1998–9.
3 Williamson LM, Lowe S, Love EM, *et al.* Serious hazards of transfusion (SHOT) initiative: analysis of the first two annual reports. *BMJ* 1999;**319**:16–19.
4 Silliman CC, Paterson AJ, Dickey WO, *et al.* The association of biologically-active lipids with the development of transfusion-related acute lung injury: a retrospective study. *Transfusion* 1997;**37**:719–26.
5 Silliman CC. Transfusion-related acute lung injury. *Transfusion Med Rev* 1999;**13**:177–86.
6 Popovsky MA. Transfusion-related acute lung injury. *Curr Opin Hematol* 2000;**7**:402–7.
7 Dry SM, Bechard KM, Milford EL, Churchill WH, Benjamin RJ. The pathology of transfusion-related acute lung injury. *Am J Clin Pathol* 1999;**112**:216–21.
8 Baudouin SV. Improved survival in ARDS: chance, technology or experience? *Thorax* 1998;**53**:237–8.
9 Wyncoll DL, Evans TW. Acute respiratory distress syndrome. *Lancet* 1999;**354**:497–501.
10 Pittet JF, Mackersie RC, Martin TR, Matthay MA. Biological markers of acute lung injury: prognostic and pathogenetic significance. *Am J Respir Crit Care Med* 1997;**155**:1187–205.
11 Ware LB, Matthay MA. The acute respiratory distress syndrome. *N Engl J Med* 2000;**342**:1334–49.
12 Gilliland HE, Armstrong MA, McMurray TJ. Tumour necrosis factor as predictor for pulmonary dysfunction after cardiac surgery. *Lancet* 1998;**352**:1281–2.

13 Dooren MC, Ouwehand WH, Verhoeven AJ, dem Borne AE, Kuijpers RW. Adult respiratory distress syndrome after experimental intravenous gamma-globulin concentrate and monocyte-reactive IgG antibodies. *Lancet* 1998;**352**:1601–2.
14 Van Buren NL, Stronek DF, Clay ME, McCullough J, Dalmasso AP. Transfusion-related acute lung injury caused by an NB2 granulocyte-specific antibody in a patient with thrombotic thrombocytopenic purpura. *Transfusion* 1990;**30**:42–5.
15 Lubenko A, Brough S, Garner S. The incidence of granulocyte antibodies in female blood donors: results of screening by a flow cytometric technique. *Platelets* 1994;**5**:234–5.
16 Hudson LD, Steinberg KP. Epidemiology of acute lung injury and ARDS. *Chest* 1999;**116**:74S–82S.

6: The use of colloids in the critically ill

CLAUDIO MARTIN

Introduction

The importance of an adequate circulating volume in the critically ill is well established. Colloids are widely used in the replacement of fluid volume, although doubts remain as to their benefits. Different colloids vary in their molecular weight and therefore in the length of time they remain in the circulatory system. Because of this and their other characteristics, they may differ in their safety and efficacy. Human albumin solutions are available for use in the emergency treatment of shock and other conditions where restoration of blood volume is urgent, and also in patients with burns and hypoproteinaemia. Plasma, albumin, synthetic colloids and crystalloids may all be used for volume expansion but the first two are expensive and crystalloids have to be given in much larger volumes than colloids to achieve the same effect. Synthetic colloids provide a cheaper, safe, effective alternative. There are three classes of synthetic colloid: dextrans, gelatins and hydroxyethyl starches. Each is available in several formulations with different properties which affect their initial plasma expanding effects, retention in the circulation and side-effects. This chapter describes the physiology of fluids and colloids, presents key animal studies that have contributed to the colloid–crystalloid debate, and describes the present clinical position.

Interstitial fluid

Interstitial fluid is essentially a gel composed of hyaluronic acid, water, proteins and ions. The primary determinant of tonicity and osmolarity is sodium concentration, along with plasma proteins – albumin and gamma globulins – which determine the plasma colloid oncotic pressure, and thus maintain adequate plasma volume. The capillary endothelium is freely permeable to small molecules but not to large protein molecules. Albumin does not therefore pass easily into the interstitial fluid despite the significant concentration gradient, due to its relatively large size compared with electrolytes. Plasma proteins, especially albumin are thus largely confined to the intravascular fluid and contribute to the colloid osmotic pressure, which opposes fluid filtration across the capillary membrane as a result of hydrostatic pressure in the vascular system.

Fluid interchange between the intravascular and interstitial fluid occurs at the capillary membrane; the main determinants of fluid movement are the Starling forces – where fluid movement is proportional to the difference between the hydrostatic and osmotic pressure gradients across the capillary wall. The reflection coefficient indicates the capillary permeability to albumin, which can vary between tissues.

Maintenance and restoration of intravascular volume are essential tasks of critical care management to achieve sufficient organ function and to avoid multiple organ failure in critically ill patients. Inadequate intravascular volume followed by impaired renal perfusion is the predominant cause of acute renal failure. There are a large number of intravenous fluid preparations available including blood, blood products, crystalloids and colloids. There has been considerable controversy as to the optimum choice of fluid replacement in any particular clinical situation.

Early restoration of circulating volume is more important in the early stages of resuscitation than the type of fluid. Crystalloids are isotonic and rapidly distribute throughout the extracellular fluid, such that large volumes are required to expand the intravascular compartment and oedema may be a problem. The large molecules contained in colloid solutions are retained within the intravascular space only if the capillary membrane is intact. The duration of effect of colloids depends upon molecule size, overall osmotic effect and plasma half-life. Albumin at 4·5% is iso-oncotic, but 20% albumin provides high colloid osmotic pressure and on infusion expands the intravascular fluid by five times the volume given by drawing fluid from the interstitial space. However, the intravascular persistence of exogenous albumin varies due to leakage into the interstitial space.

Colloid versus crystalloid?

The optimal composition of fluid for volume resuscitation in critically ill patients has been the subject of controversy for decades.[1-4] Clinicians are faced with several options, including crystalloid solutions of varying tonicity, several colloid preparations (albumin and others), and blood products. Some of these solutions may be differentially distributed between the intra- and extra-vascular, and intra- and extra-cellular compartments, accounting for a variety of physiological effects. The argument in favour of crystalloids is based on the fact that acute changes in blood volume and extracellular fluid can easily be corrected. However, administration of large volumes may be required to maintain the plasma volume and expansion of the interstitial fluid is likely, resulting in oedema. In favour of colloids is that these provide a better haemodynamic response and plasma volume expansion and most remain in the circulation – provided capillary permeability is intact. However, colloids can leak from the circulation in critically ill patients when capillary integrity is lost.

Crystalloid solutions supply water and sodium to maintain the osmotic gradient between the extravascular and intravascular compartments. Examples are lactated Ringer's solution and 0·9% sodium chloride. Colloidal solutions, such as those containing albumin, dextrans, or starches, increase the plasma oncotic pressure and effectively move fluid from the interstitial compartment to the plasma compartment. Oxygen-carrying resuscitation fluids, such as whole blood and artificial haemoglobin solutions, not only increase plasma volume but improve tissue oxygenation. Clinically, colloidal solutions are generally superior to crystalloids in their ability to expand plasma volume. However, colloids may impair coagulation, interfere with organ function, and cause anaphylactoid reactions. Crystalloid solutions represent the least expensive option and are less likely to promote bleeding, but they are more likely to cause oedema because larger volumes are needed. Perhaps more importantly, crystalloid solutions are much cheaper, particularly compared to blood products such as albumin. A cost-effectiveness analysis comparing colloidal and crystalloidal fluid for resuscitation efforts was reported by Bisonni et al. in 1991,[4] and revealed no statistically significant differences in mortality rates. The cost of each life saved using crystalloids was $45·13, and the cost of each life saved using colloidal solutions was a massive $1493·60.

Animal studies

Animal studies have provided useful evidence of the relative benefits or otherwise of colloid versus crystalloids. Morisaki and co-workers[5] tested the hypothesis that the type of fluid infused to chronically maintain intravascular volumes would modify both microvascular integrity and cellular structure in extrapulmonary organs in hyperdynamic sepsis. They used an awake sheep caecal ligation and perforation model of sepsis. Sheep were treated for 48 hours with either 10% pentastarch (n=9), 10% pentafraction (n=8), or Ringer's lactate (n=8), titrated to maintain a constant left atrial pressure. Biopsy samples were then taken from the left ventricle and gastrocnemius muscle for electron microscopy.

The volume required to maintain the left atrial pressure in animals randomised to receive crystalloid was 11 062 ml over 48 hours compared to only 2845 ml in the sheep which received colloid. All animals had similar hyperdynamic circulatory responses and increased systemic oxygen utilisation and organ blood flow. However, the capillary luminal areas with less endothelial swelling were lower and less parenchymal injury was found in sheep treated with pentastarch compared to Ringer's lactate infusion in both muscle types. Pentafraction showed no benefits over pentastarch. The authors concluded that chronic intravascular volume resuscitation of hyperdynamic sepsis with pentastarch in this sheep model blunted the progression of both microvascular and parenchymal injury, and suggested that microvascular surface area for tissue oxygen exchange in sepsis may be better preserved with colloid, resulting in less parenchymal injury.[5] The reduction in myocardium morphological injury score as a result of pentastarch administration compared to Ringer's lactate is shown in Figure 6.1. Each micrograph is scored on the overall cellular injury, mitochondrial injury, oedema, glycogen stores and nuclear change. For each of these parameters it is clear that the colloid treated animals had significantly less cellular injury in the myocardium compared to the crystalloid treated animals. The same also applied to skeletal muscle.

The question remains – do these structural and morphological changes translate into functional changes in those organs?

In a study from this author's laboratory which has not yet been published, a caecal ligation and puncture sepsis model of rats was used. Animals were randomised to resuscitation with either albumin (2·5 ml/kg/hour) or saline (10 ml/kg/hour) for 24 hours. The values of central venous pressure, mean arterial pressure, cardiac index, arterial lactate and oxygen saturation did

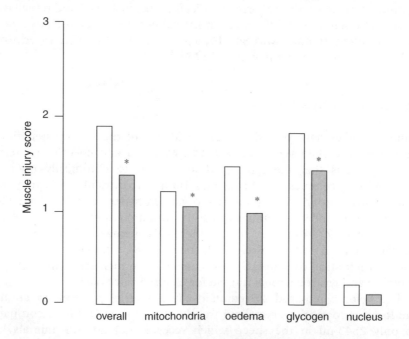

Figure 6.1 Myocardial tissue injury scores in a sheep model of sepsis. Animals were resuscitated with either Ringer's lactate (open bars) or pentastarch (grey bars). Each micrograph was scored on the overall cellular injury, mitochondrial injury, oedema, glycogen stores and nuclear change. Bars are mean scores and asterisks indicate $p < 0.05$ between treatment groups. Reproduced from Morisaki H, et al. J Appl Physiol 1994;77:1507–18[5] with permission from Springer–Verlag.

not differ between groups. The two modes of resuscitation resulted therefore in equivalent haemodynamic responses in septic rats. Organ function in terms of kidney, gut and myocardium was also studied. Glomerular filtration rate and tubular function in terms of the fractional excretion of sodium were not different, and neither was urinary protein excretion.

Translocation of bacteria and endotoxin during sepsis may be mediated in part by bowel mucosal microcirculatory dysfunction. Gut function was therefore investigated in two different ways in animals resuscitated with either albumin or saline. The first was investigation of gut perfusion using intravital microscopy with the gut mucosa exposed to study the mucosal circulation. This technique was originally described by Farqhuar et al.[6] where laser Doppler measurements of bowel wall blood flow and intravital microscopy of the mucosal microcirculation was undertaken. The areas surrounded by perfused capillaries (intercapillary area) were then measured using video analysis software. Laser Doppler flowmetry revealed a decrease in bowel wall blood flow in the non-septic rats, which did not occur in the septic animals. The intercapillary areas were significantly greater in the septic compared to non-septic rats.[6] Sepsis induced by caecal ligation and puncture therefore leads to a decrease in the number of perfused capillaries in the small bowel mucosa.

Another study using a similar sepsis model in rats investigated whether normotensive sepsis affects the ability of the microcirculation to appropriately regulate microregional red blood cell flux.[7] Using intravital microscopy of an extensor digitorum longus muscle preparation, it was shown that sepsis was associated with a 36% reduction in perfused capillary density and a 265% increase in stopped-flow capillaries; the spatial distribution of perfused capillaries was also 72% more heterogeneous. Mean intercapillary distance increased by 30% in the septic animals. However, when the intercapillary distance was compared between animals resuscitated with albumin or saline,[8] there was no difference between the two groups.

The second aspect of gut function that was studied in the septic rat model was mucosal permeability, measured using radio-labelled ethylene diamine tetra acetic acid (EDTA). The EDTA is injected intravenously and its appearance monitored in a perfused segment of the ileum. Because EDTA diffuses freely from the plasma space to the interstitial space its appearance in the gut lumen represents permeability of the mucosa. However since there are changes in gut perfusion that might alter the delivery of the EDTA to the mucosa, urea is also injected, which is freely diffusible through the gut mucosa. The appearance of urea in the luminal perfusate is therefore a measure of gut perfusion to the mucosa. Hence the ratio of EDTA to urea in the gut lumen is a measure of mucosal permeability. In the septic rat model, animals with sepsis have an increase in the EDTA/urea ratio i.e. indicating an increase in gut mucosal permeability. However, again there is no difference between animals resuscitated with albumin compared to saline.[8]

Myocardial function was also investigated using the caecal ligation and perforation rat model of sepsis described above. An isolated heart Langdorf preparation was used. The myocardial contractility and an increase in preload appeared to be better, but this finding was not statistically significant. The left ventricular recovery of isolated Langdorf preparations from ischaemic insult was also studied. Animals were subjected to 60 minutes of warm ischaemia and recovery was monitored at 30 and 60 minutes. There was no difference between animals which received albumin compared to those which received saline. Lung tissue was also collected and myeloperoxidase activity and F2 isoprostane as a measure of oxidant stress were also not different irrespective of whether rats were treated with albumin or saline. These data suggest no benefit of albumin over saline for the resuscitation of sepsis in terms of organ function.

Thus the studies using the sheep model[5] apparently contradict the findings in the rat model. In sheep there was apparently a benefit of the colloid pentastarch in terms of structural injury but experiments with the rat model with albumin shows no functional advantage.

Clinical studies

The two Cochrane reviews, which have been recently updated, reported on colloid solutions for resuscitation[9] and colloids versus crystalliod.[10] The report by Bunn et al.[9] compared the effects of different colloid solutions in patients thought to need volume replacement since different colloids vary in their molecular weight and therefore in the length of time they remain in the circulatory system. Because of this and their other characteristics, they may differ in their safety and efficacy. Fifty-two trials met the inclusion criteria, with a total of 3311 patients. For albumin or plasma protein fraction (PPF) versus hydroxyethyl starch (HES) 20 trials (n = 1029) reported mortality. The pooled relative risk was 1·17 (95% CI 0·91–1·50). For albumin or PPF versus gelatine four trials (n = 542) reported mortality. The pooled relative risk was 0·99 (0·69–1·42). For gelatine versus HES six trials (n = 597) reported mortality and the relative risk was 0·96 (0·69–1·33). Relative risk was not estimable in the albumin versus dextran, gelatine versus dextran, and HES versus dextran groups. In 15 trials adverse reactions were recorded, but in the event no such adverse reactions actually occurred. From this review, there is no evidence that one colloid solution is more effective or safe than any other, although the confidence intervals are wide and do not exclude clinically significant differences between colloids. The authors concluded that larger trials of fluid therapy are needed to detect or exclude clinically significant differences in mortality.

The second report by the same authors[10] reported on the effect of human albumin and PPF administration in the management of critically ill patients, on mortality. Randomised controlled trials comparing albumin/PPF with no albumin/PPF, or with a crystalloid solution, in critically ill patients with hypovolaemia, burns or hypoalbuminaemia were included. Thirty trials met the inclusion criteria and there were 156 deaths among 1419 patients. For each patient category the risk of death in the albumin treated group was higher than in the comparison group. The pooled relative risk of death with albumin administration was 1·68 (1·26–2·23). Overall, the risk of death in patients receiving albumin was 14% compared to 8% in the control groups, an increase in the risk of death of 6% (3%–9%). These data suggest that for every 17 critically ill patient treated with albumin there is one additional death. It was concluded that there is no evidence that albumin administration reduces the risk of death in critically ill patients with hypovolaemia, burns or hypoalbuminaemia, and in contrast a strong suggestion that it may increase the risk of death.

The validity of the studies included in these reviews has of course been questioned extensively. A variety of serious limitations apply, suggesting that their findings be interpreted cautiously. Webb[11] reviewed the Cochrane reports[9,10] and stated that more than half of the randomised controlled trials included were reported prior to 1990 and hence did not reflect current practice. Trials included were heterogeneous with respect to patient characteristics, type of illness, administered fluids and physiological endpoints. Differences in illness severity, concomitant therapies and fluid management approaches were not taken into account. Very few trials were blinded. The author concluded that the Cochrane report did not support the conclusion that choice of resuscitation fluid is a major determinant of mortality in critically ill patients, or that changes to current fluid management practice are required. Changes such as exclusive reliance on crystalloids would necessitate a reassessment of the goals and methods of fluid therapy. Since the effect on mortality may be minimal or non-existent, this author concluded that choice of resuscitation fluid should rest on whether the particular fluid permits the intensive care unit to provide better patient care.

It is possible that delivery of the colloid may be improved, and bolus therapy may be better than continuous infusion. Ernest and colleagues[12] determined the relative distribution of fluid within the extracellular fluid volume (ECFV) after infusing either normal saline or 5% albumin in septic, critically ill patients in a prospective, randomised, unblinded study. Eighteen septic, critically ill patients were randomised to infusion of either normal saline or 5% albumin to a haemodynamic end point determined by the patient's clinician. Plasma volume, ECFV, cardiac index, and arterial oxygen content were measured immediately before (baseline) and after each fluid infusion. Plasma volume and ECFV were measured by dilution of ^{131}I labelled albumin and ^{35}S labelled sodium sulphate, respectively. Interstitial fluid volume (ISFV) was calculated as ECFV − plasma volume. Baseline values for plasma, ISFV, ECFV, and oxygen delivery index did not differ between treatment groups. Infusion of normal saline increased the ECFV by approximately the volume infused, and the expansion of the plasma volume to ISFV was in a ratio of 1:3. Infusion of 5% albumin increased the ECFV by double the volume infused, with both the plasma volume and ISFV expanding by approximately equal amounts. Oxygen delivery index did not increase after either infusion due to the effect of haemodilution. Expansion of the ECFV in excess of the volume of 5% albumin infused suggests that fluid may move from the intracellular fluid volume to the ECFV in septic patients who receive this fluid.

The question for future experiments is what are appropriate endpoints – do we really expect that our fluid therapy is going to alter mortality or would we be better looking at an intermediate outcome such as haemodynamics, fluid balance and organ function. These are all questions to consider – the question of colloid versus crystalloid remains unresolved. Despite the Cochrane reviews, many clinicians still believe intuitively that colloids, including albumin, have a role in medical practice and continue to use them.

Summary

There is no ideal colloid but those with low molecular weights such as gelatins are more suitable for rapid, short term volume expansion whilst in states of capillary leak where longer term effects are required hydroxyethyl starches are more effective. Dextrans are as effective as the alternatives but produce more side-effects and the need to pre-treat with hapten-dextran renders them unwieldy in use. Albumin is as persistent as hydroxyethyl starch in the healthy circulation but is retained less well in states of capillary leak. Human albumin solutions are more expensive than other colloids and crystalloids.

Key questions remain unresolved regarding the advantages and limitations of colloids for fluid resuscitation despite extensive investigation. Elucidation of these questions has been slowed, in part, by uncertainty as to the optimal endpoints that should be monitored in assessing patient response to administered fluid. Crystalloids currently serve as the first-line fluids in hypovolaemic patients. Colloids can be considered in patients with severe or acute shock or hypovolaemia resulting from sudden plasma loss. Colloids may be combined with crystalloids to obviate administration of large crystalloid volumes. Further clinical trials are needed to define the optimal role for colloids in critically ill patients.

References

1   Ross AD, Angaran DM. Colloids vs. crystalloids – a continuing controversy. *Drug Intell Clin Pharm* 1984;**18**:202–12.

2   Shoemaker WC. Hemodynamic and oxygen transport effects of crystalloids and colloids in critically ill patients. *Curr Stud Hematol Blood Transfus* 1986;**53**:155–76.

3   Davies MJ. Crystalloid or colloid: does it matter? *J Clin Anesth* 1989;**1**:464–71.

4   Bisonni RS, Holtgrave DR, Lawler F, Marley DS. Colloids versus crystalloids in fluid resuscitation: an analysis of randomized controlled trials. *J Fam Pract* 1991;**32**:387–90.

5   Morisaki H, Bloos F, Keys J, Martin C, Neal A, Sibbald WJ. Compared with crystalloid, colloid therapy slows progression of extrapulmonary tissue injury in septic sheep. *J Appl Physiol* 1994;**77**:1507–18.

6   Farquhar I, Martin CM, Lam C, Potter R, Ellis CG, Sibbald WJ. Decreased capillary density **in vivo** in bowel mucosa of rats with normotensive sepsis. *J Surg Res* 1996;**61**:190–6.

7   Lam C, Tyml K, Martin C, Sibbald W. Microvascular perfusion is impaired in a rat model of normotensive sepsis. *J Clin Invest* 1994;**94**:2077–83.

8   Tham LCH, Yu P, Punnen S, Martin CM. Comparison of the effects of albumin and crystalloid infusions on gut microcirculation in normotensive septic rats. *Am J Respir Crit Care Med* 2001;**163**:A556 (Abstract).

9   Bunn F, Alderson P, Hawkins V. Colloid solutions for fluid resuscitation (Cochrane Review). *Cochrane Database Syst Rev* 2001;**2**:CD001319.

10 Bunn F, Lefebvre C, Li Wan Po A, Li L, Roberts I, Schierhout G. Human albumin solution for resuscitation and volume expansion in critically ill patients. The Albumin Reviewers. *Cochrane Database Syst Rev* 2000;**2**:CD001208.

11 Webb AR. The appropriate role of colloids in managing fluid imbalance: a critical review of recent meta-analytic findings. *Crit Care* 2000;**4 Suppl 2**: S26–32.

12 Ernest D, Belzberg AS, Dodek PM. Distribution of normal saline and 5% albumin infusions in septic patients. *Crit Care Med* 1999;**27**:46–50.

7: Radical reactions of haem proteins

CHRIS E COOPER

Introduction

This article will provide an overview of basic free radical chemistry and biology before focusing on the reactions of haemoglobin and myoglobin as sources of free radical damage. Finally, the clinical relevance of such globin molecules in pathology will be discussed, with particular emphasis on the processes involved in rhabdomyolysis and the possible toxic effects of novel haemoglobin based blood substitutes.

Free radical chemistry

Atoms consist of a nucleus (made up of uncharged neutrons and positively charged protons) surrounded by negatively charged electrons in defined orbitals. Each orbital can accept two electrons with different spins; the majority of biological molecules have all their orbitals full of such paired electrons. Each of the electrons has an opposite spin and therefore most biological molecules contain no overall electron spin. Free radicals are atoms or molecules containing an odd number of electrons, such that one (or more) is unpaired. This results in an uncompensated spin. As a moving spin creates a magnetic field, species with unpaired electrons (denoted thus $^\bullet$) are termed paramagnetic (and if these species are aligned macroscopically then their paramagnetism is responsible for the bulk of the magnetism we observe in everyday life).

More important for biology and medicine is that many free radicals are very reactive species, since they endeavour to fill this unfilled electron orbital. For example, molecular oxygen has two unpaired electrons in its outer orbital and is therefore paramagnetic. The reduction of oxygen to water requires four electrons that have to be added one at a time.

$$O_2 + e^- \longrightarrow O_2^{-\bullet} + e^- \longrightarrow O_2^{2-} + e^- \longrightarrow OH^\bullet + e^- \longrightarrow H_2O$$

Oxygen $\qquad$ superoxide $\qquad$ peroxide $\qquad$ hydroxyl $\qquad$ water
$\qquad\qquad\qquad\qquad\qquad\qquad\qquad\qquad\qquad\qquad$ radical

Of the three intermediates in this process two are free radicals (superoxide and hydroxyl radicals) and the third (peroxide) has a tendency to generate free radicals in reactions as discussed later in this article. The four-electron reduction of oxygen occurs in the mitochondrial electron transport system of all aerobically respiring cells. The enzyme which catalyses this reaction (cytochrome c oxidase) contains the transition metals iron and copper in its active site. These ions can be paramagnetic and contain stable unpaired electrons in their d-orbitals. By using the unpaired electrons in these transition metals to control the oxygen reactions, mitochondria prevent the unwanted release of oxygen-derived free radicals.[1]

Reactions of free radicals

Although free radical reactions are generally considered detrimental, it has long been known that enzymes use the reactivity of free radicals to catalyse biological chemistry, for example, respiration, thyroid hormone synthesis, prostaglandin metabolism and DNA synthesis, to name but a few. More recently signalling roles have been discovered for free radicals. Therefore the perception that formation of free radicals *in vivo* necessarily represents a pathological event is changing to encompass the idea that these reactive species can in fact regulate numerous physiological processes. The classic example is the free radical nitric oxide, which has diverse physiological roles in the vasculature, in host immune responses and in the nervous system.[2] Nitric oxide stimulation of soluble guanylate cyclase in the vascular smooth muscle activates a signalling cascade that eventually leads to relaxation of the vessel or, in platelets, to an inhibition of aggregation. These properties of nitric oxide have defined key roles for this free radical in the mechanisms that maintain vascular homeostasis.

However, one should not neglect the "dark side" of free radical reactivity. A number of biological processes have the ability to generate unstable reactive oxygen and nitrogen based free radicals (Box 7.1).

Polyunsaturated fatty acids are particularly vulnerable to free radical attack by the process of hydrogen abstraction (removal of a hydrogen atom), causing lipid peroxidation and decreased membrane fluidity. Oxygen-derived free radical damage to proteins can result in fragmentation, cross-linking, aggregation and consequent loss of enzyme activity. Nitric oxide can nitrate proteins (probably mediated indirectly via peroxynitrite or $NO_2^{\bullet}$ intermediates) and hence affect enzyme activity.

Iron and free radicals

Hydroxyl radical formation

Free ferrous iron in solution has the ability to generate toxic free radicals. In the presence of peroxide, for example, Fenton chemistry generates the

---

Box 7.1 Free radicals

Oxygen based free radicals

- hydroxyl $OH^{\bullet}$
- superoxide $O_2^{-\bullet}$
- peroxyl $ROO^{\bullet}$
- alkoxyl $RO^{\bullet}$
- hydroperoxyl $RHOO^{\bullet}$

Nitrogen based free radicals

- nitric oxide $NO^{\bullet}$
- nitrogen dioxide $NO_2^{\bullet}$

---

hydroxyl radical ($OH^{\bullet}$):

$$Fe^{2+} + H_2O_2 \longrightarrow Fe^{3+} + OH^- + OH^{\bullet}$$

The hydroxyl radical is so reactive that its lifetime is in effect only as long as the distance to the first molecule it collides with. Therefore its average diffusion distance is $<5\text{Å}$. This intense reactivity has a number of corollaries, not always appreciated by biomedical researchers: biology has utilised molecules for iron metabolism (haem proteins), storage (ferritin) and transport (transferrin) that lock the iron in a state where Fenton chemistry cannot occur. Hydroxyl radicals formed by Fenton chemistry react where they are formed, i.e. they cannot diffuse to a distant site and cause an effect.

Although it is possible to use scavengers to detect the presence of hydroxyl radicals, it not possible to use them to prevent the biological effects. Because $OH^{\bullet}$ reacts with all biomolecules at diffusion limited rates, a scavenger would need to be present at essentially the same concentration as the total of all cellular biomolecules to prevent its biological reactivity. Therefore studies using so-called hydroxyl radical scavengers (for example, mannitol) to prevent $OH^{\bullet}$ reactivity are fundamentally flawed.[3] Any biological effects observed cannot be via trapping a significant amount of $OH^{\bullet}$. Instead the way forward in preventing Fenton chemistry is to stop iron (or copper which has similar reactivity) being available in a form that can catalyse the reaction.

Haem protein radical formation

Iron can exist in a number of redox states, differing by the addition or subtraction of an electron: ferrous (Fe^{2+}), ferric (Fe^{3+}) and ferryl (Fe^{4+}).

Many ferric haem proteins react with peroxide to form ferryl haem and a protein bound free radical [4]:

$$Fe^{3+} + H_2O_2 + R \longrightarrow Fe^{4+} = O_2^- + H_2O + R^{\bullet+}$$
(R represents the rest of the protein)

As stated previously a wide variety of enzymes stabilise free radicals as reactive intermediates, necessary to drive catalysis. In particular haem iron-containing enzymes involved in biosynthesis (for example, thyroid peroxidase and prostaglandin H synthase) or in host defence (for example, catalase, myeloperoxidase and lactoperoxidase) are activated by hydrogen peroxide to generate reactive free radicals bound to the protein (Figure 7.1). Problems can arise when ferryl iron and free radicals are generated in proteins not designed to control this activity. In particular the reaction of hydrogen peroxide with globins in the ferric state can result in the formation of strongly oxidising radicals able to initiate cellular damage.

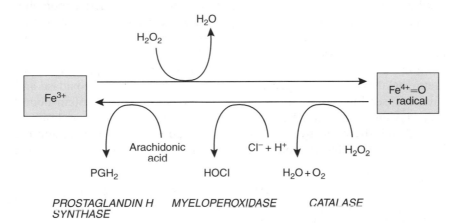

Figure 7.1 The reactions of ferryl iron and haem radicals in defence and biosynthesis. Catalases and peroxidases have a common first reaction with peroxide that generates two strong oxidants: ferryl haem and a protein-bound free radical. The subsequent reactivity of these species then differs depending on the specific enzyme. This diversity is seen in the three examples illustrated: enzymes involved in detoxification (catalase), defence (myeloperoxidase) and biosynthesis (prostaglandin H synthase).

Haemoglobin and myoglobin redox states

The normal redox state of haemoglobin and myoglobin is ferrous iron (Fe^{2+}), which will reversibly bind oxygen to form a stable oxy complex (oxyhaemoglobin). However, the oxy complex has the potential to autoxidise to form the ferric (met) haemoglobin and superoxide radical (Figure 7.2).

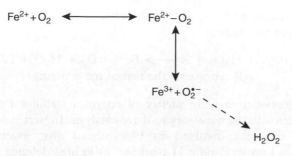

Figure 7.2 Haemoglobin and myoglobin redox states. Ferrous haemoglobin/myoglobin reversibly binds oxygen. A spontaneous "autoxidation" rate generates the ferric(met) species and the superoxide radical. The latter can react either spontaneously, or in the presence of the enzyme superoxide dismutase, to form hydrogen peroxide.

The superoxide formed can then further react to form peroxide and this will contribute to oxidative stress, either by reacting with haemoglobin itself (see below) or other cellular targets. Methaemoglobin cannot bind oxygen, until re-converted to the ferrous species by the enzyme methaemoglobin reductase. However, the loss of oxygen binding capacity by the formation of methaemoglobin is not a major problem; what is of concern is its reactivity with peroxide.

Figure 7.3 shows the reaction between methaemoglobin (or metmyoglobin) and hydrogen peroxide. As in the case of peroxidase and catalases (see Figure 7.1) the products are ferryl iron and a protein-bound radical. Unlike the peroxidases/catalases, however, globins are not designed to deal with these reactive species. Both the globin-bound radical and the highly oxidative ferryl iron can cause oxidative stress by generating

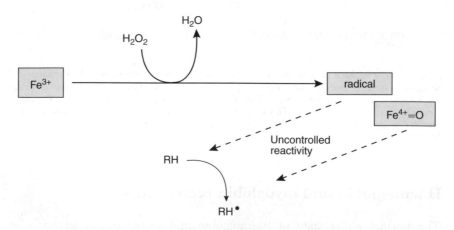

Figure 7.3 Haemoglobin and myoglobin radicals. The reactions of the methaemoglobin/myoglobin and the peroxide formed in Figure 7.2 results in the same oxidative products as in the peroxidases/catalase system (Figure 7.1). However, there is no control over the subsequent reactivity and both the ferryl iron and the globin radicals can initiate free radical damage.

secondary free radical products. Redox cycling between the ferric and ferryl forms of haem proteins can initiate lipid peroxidation and other free radical mediated reactions.[5]

We can detect ferryl haemoglobin by optical spectroscopy both *in vitro* and *in vivo* (Figure 7.4). The globin-bound free radicals can be studied using the technique of electron paramagnetic resonance (EPR). This detects the paramagnetism of the unpaired electron and is the only technique that directly enables identification and quantitation of free radical species. The EPR spectra of the globin radical in whole blood is shown in Figure 7.5.[6]

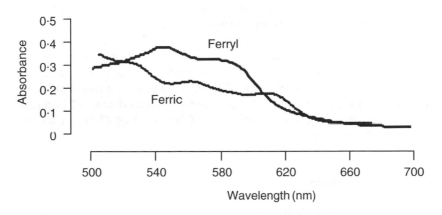

Figure 7.4 Optical spectrum of ferryl haemoglobin. The visible spectra of haemoglobin in the ferric (met) and ferryl forms are distinguishable. The ferryl spectrum was obtained by adding 100 μM hydrogen peroxide to 50 μM methaemoglobin.

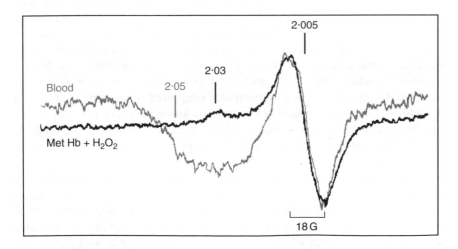

Figure 7.5 Electron paramagnetic resonance identification of haem radicals in blood. The EPR spectrum of whole blood from a healthy donor is compared to that of ferryl haemoglobin. The signal at g = 2·005 is a tyrosine radical and is identical whether measured in whole blood or following the addition of 1 mM hydrogen peroxide to 100 μM purified methaemoglobin. Spectra are redrawn from data presented in Svistunenko DA, et al. J Biol Chem 1997;272:7114–21.[6]

71

Clinical relevance of ferric/ferryl redox cycling

There are several clinical conditions where the globin ferric/ferryl redox cycle may become pathologically relevant.[5] These include ischaemia and reperfusion, where ferryl myoglobin may help initiate myocardial injury; in the brain ferryl haemoglobin may damage arteries in subarachnoid haemorrhage; in stroke the modified haemoglobin has the potential to cross the blood–brain barrier. In addition, any situation where haemolysis occurs removes haemoglobin from within the protective environment of the red blood cell membrane and therefore unleashes its potential for initiating free radical damage. Such situations clinically include sickle cell or haemolytic anaemia and even atherosclerosis. In order to study the clinical effects in more detail we have focused on the two main conditions where there are high level of ferric haem proteins outside the cell: rhabdomyolysis (myoglobin)[7] and during the use of haemoglobin based blood substitutes (haemoglobin).[8] The topic of rhabdomyolysis is also discussed in terms of the mechanism of acute renal failure in Chapter 3 of *Critical Care Focus Volume 1 (Renal Failure)*.[9]

Rhabdomyolysis

In the United States, rhabdomyolysis accounts for 7% of all cases of acute renal failure, as a result of massive muscle breakdown caused predominantly by trauma, but also by hypothermia, seizures, muscle ischaemia and alcohol or drug abuse. The muscle breakdown leads to release of myoglobin from muscle cells into the circulation; myoglobin then accumulates in the kidney in the ferric Fe^{3+} state. Renal vasoconstriction follows in a process associated with free radical production. Thirty per cent of patients with significant rhabdomyolysis can go on to develop renal failure, both as a result of tubular obstruction, and via vasoconstriction-mediated tubular necrosis. Treatment by alkalinisation was suggested to work by solubilising myoglobin to prevent tubular obstruction; however, there is no evidence that myoglobin solubility is increased following alkalinisation. Instead we have recently determined that raising the pH prevents the oxidative-stress inducing reactions of myoglobin.[10]

In animal models of rhabdomyolysis, animals are treated with glycerol, which causes massive muscle breakdown and mimics human rhabdomyolysis. Morphological examination shows a massive deposition of metmyoglobin in the kidney. Optical spectroscopy of the kidneys identifies the characteristic band of metmyoglobin at 630 nm, but also shows the presence of oxidatively modified haem proteins (Figure 7.6). Modified haem is also present in the urine of patients with rhabdomyolysis.[11]

Electron paramagnetic resonance, as well as being able to detect free radicals, can also detect unpaired electrons in transition metals. The ferric

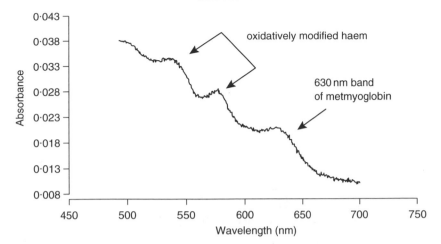

Figure 7.6 Optical spectrum of rhabdomyolytic kidney. The visible spectrum of an extract of myoglobin from a rat treated with glycerol to induce rhabdomyolysis. Spectral features characteristic of metmyoglobin and oxidatively damaged myoglobin haem are indicated. Spectra are redrawn from data presented in Moore KP, et al. J Biol Chem 1998;273:31731–37. [10]

state of iron, such as is present in metmyoglobin, is very easy to detect and accurately quantitate by this technique. In the study by Moore *et al.*,[10] glycerol treatment induced oxidant injury in the kidney; myoglobin-induced lipid peroxidation caused a 30-fold increase in the formation of F_2-isoprostanes, which are potent renal vasoconstrictors. Urinary excretion of F_2-isoprostanes also increased compared to controls. Administration of alkali improved renal function and significantly reduced the urinary excretion of F_2-isoprostanes by approximately 80%. Electron paramagnetic resonance confirmed that myoglobin was deposited in the kidneys as the redox active ferric (met)myoglobin; the amount of metmyoglobin in the kidney was unaffected by alkalinisation, i.e. no increase in solubilisation was observed. However, kinetic studies demonstrated that the reactivity of ferryl myoglobin, which is responsible for inducing lipid peroxidation, was reduced at alkaline pH. Myoglobin-induced lipid peroxidation was also inhibited at alkaline pH. The effect of pH on the stability of ferryl myoglobin, lipid peroxidation and isoprostane formation is shown in Figure 7.7.[10,12]

These data strongly support a causative role for oxidative injury in the mechanism of renal failure following rhabdomyolysis and suggest that the protective effect of alkalinisation is a result of inhibition of myoglobin-induced lipid peroxidation and consequent isoprostane induced vasoconstriction. In effect the addition of alkalinisation turns a vicious cycle into a virtuous one. Myoglobin-induced F_2-isoprostane formation induces vasoconstriction and associated ischaemia which decreases the pH; at a lower pH myoglobin is more reactive and therefore even more isoprostanes are formed and there is increased vasoconstriction etc. On

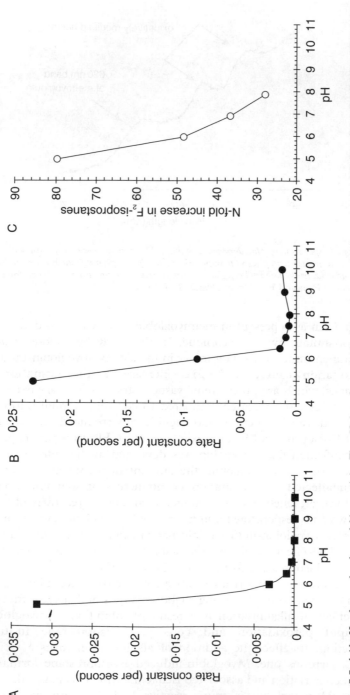

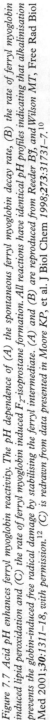

Figure 7.7 *Acid pH enhances ferryl myoglobin reactivity. The pH dependence of (A) the spontaneous ferryl myoglobin decay rate, (B) the rate of ferryl myoglobin induced lipid peroxidation and (C) the rate of ferryl myoglobin induced F_2-isoprostane formation. All reactions have identical pH profiles indicating that alkalinisation prevents the globin-induced free radical damage by stabilising the ferryl intermediate. (A) and (B) are reproduced from Reeder BJ, and Wilson MT, Free Rad Biol Med 2001;30:1311–18, with permission.[12] (C) is redrawn from data presented in Moore KP, et al. J Biol Chem 1998;273:31731–7.[10]*

the other hand by increasing the pH, following the addition of alkali, myoglobin reactivity is reduced; this decreases the rate of formation of F_2-isoprostanes and therefore causes vasodilatation, this in turn reduces the ischaemia and raises the pH further, resulting in decreased myoglobin reactivity etc.

Haemoglobin based blood substitutes

Haemoglobin based blood substitutes are designed to be used in emergencies or during surgery when rapid expansion of the blood volume with an oxygen carrier is needed.[8,13] The two main types of products in development are based on cell-free haemoglobin or perfluorocarbon emulsions. Outside the erythrocyte haemoglobin has much too high an oxygen affinity. Also its rapid clearance from the circulation leads to renal toxicity (probably via exactly the same mechanism as myoglobin induces rhabdomyolysis). Various strategies have been used to overcome these problems including structural modification of haemoglobin or the use of recombinant technology to synthesise haemoglobin mutants. The goal of these approaches has been to produce a haemoglobin molecule with lower oxygen affinity and greater structural stability. Stabilisation of the tetrameric structure by either crosslinking covalently (for example, with diaspirin pyridoxal phosphates) polymerisation (for example, with glutaraldehyde) and/or conjugation (for example, with polyoxyethylene) increases the lifetime of cell free haemoglobin in the body and has the additional desired effect of decreasing the oxygen affinity.

However, both *in vitro* and *in vivo* studies suggest even these modified haemoglobins have additional toxicity problems. This is highlighted by a recent clinical trial using diaspirin cross-linked haemoglobin, which has advantageous properties with respect to oxygen affinity and structural stability.[14] In this study, administration of haemoglobin increased the incidence of death in patients treated for haemorrhagic shock when compared to control patients treated with saline. Central to the proposed mechanisms underlying these findings are the reactions between haemoglobin and reactive nitrogen or oxygen species.[15] Cell free haemoglobin binds free nitric oxide (thus inducing hypertension) and has the potential to undergo ferric/ferryl redox cycling. The modified haemoglobins themselves have a tendency to undergo increased autoxidation (forming excess methaemoglobin) and outside the erythrocyte there is no catalase to lower the peroxide concentration.

Oxidant stress

Figure 7.8 demonstrates the reactivity of various modified haemoglobins to hydrogen peroxide in terms of ferryl iron formation (Figure 7.8A) and free

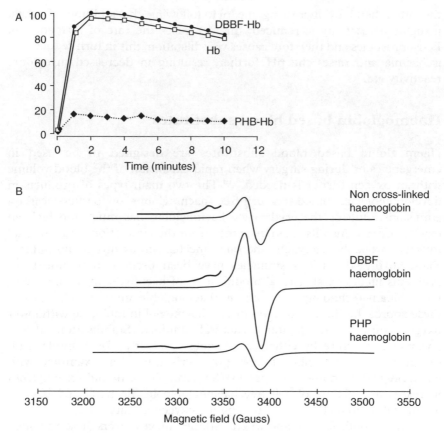

Figure 7.8 Ferryl iron and free radical formation in haemoglobin based blood substitutes. (A) The extent of ferryl formation following the addition of 100 μM hydrogen peroxide to 50 μM methaemoglobin. (B) Electron paramagnetic resonance (EPR) spectra 30 seconds after peroxide addition indicating the presence of globin-based free radicals: PHP is haemoglobin cross-linked between the lys-82 residue of one β-subunit and the N terminal of the other and then conjugated with polyoxyethylene; DBBF is haemoglobin cross-linked between the lys-99 residues of the α-subunits; non cross-linked haemoglobin is normal HbA_0. Spectra reproduced from: Dunne J, et al. Adv Exp Med Biol 1999;471:9–15[16] with permission.

radical formation (Figure 7.8B).[16] We compared PHP haemoglobin (cross-linked between the β-subunits and conjugated with polyoxyethylene) with DBBF haemoglobin (cross-linked between the β-subunits using bis(dibromosalicylfumarate)), and control HbA_0. All the blood substitutes generated ferryl haem and globin free radicals.[16] However, it can be seen that PHP haemoglobin formed less ferryl haem and less free radicals than either DBBF or control haemoglobin. This is because PHP uses a less pure form of haemoglobin as its starting material.[17] Small concentrations of "contaminating" erythrocyte catalase are present which catalyse the production of water from hydrogen peroxide. Whether this makes the product less toxic *in vivo* remains to be seen.

Nitric oxide

The reaction with oxyhaemoglobin is a major mechanism for disarming nitric oxide bioactivity in mammals.[18,19] The reaction between haemoglobin and nitric oxide is important both in the context of how nitric oxide functions *in vivo* and the biological effects of cell-free haemoglobin. In the field of blood substitutes, development of a useful agent has been thwarted to date by the problem that genetically engineered and chemically modified products invariably suffer from their ability to scavenge nitric oxide, thereby eliciting systemic hypertension.[20] The extent of the hypertensive response correlates with the rate of nitric oxide scavenging by the haem, indicating that haemoglobin modulates vessel reactivity primarily through a nitric oxide-dependent mechanism. It should be mentioned, however, that alternative mechanisms of haemoglobin-dependent hypertension have also been reported and include modulation of adrenergic receptor sensitivity and stimulation of the vasoconstrictor peptide, endothelin-1.[21,22]

A haemoglobin based oxygen carrier whose reaction with nitric oxide is significantly inhibited yet can still reversibly bind oxygen would be an ideal candidate for a blood substitute. Recombinant technology has been used to investigate the effects of mutating different amino acid residues close to the haem groups on nitric oxide binding. As well as the haem iron group reacting with nitric oxide, haemoglobin also has the potential to transport nitric oxide bound to a conserved cysteine residue on the beta-chain (RS-NO).[23] Mutating this residue may affect the nitric oxide reactivity of haemoglobin *in vivo*. Other useful strategies to limit nitric oxide scavenging include mimicking red blood cells by encapsulation of the haemoglobin into liposomes.[13]

Summary

Free radicals are implicated in many pathological conditions. Free haem proteins in the circulation can participate in radical reactions that result in toxicity. These reactions have been shown to be relevant particularly in rhabdomyolysis and the side effects of haemoglobin based blood substitutes. Clinical experiences with chemically modified and genetically engineered haemoglobin blood substitutes have uncovered side effects that must be addressed before a viable oxygen-carrying alternative to blood can be developed. Research is now being directed towards understanding the mechanisms of these toxic side effects and developing methods of overcoming them.

Acknowledgements

I am indebted to all the haemoglobin and myoglobin researchers at the University of Essex for their contribution to the work presented in this article, in particular Jackie Dunne, Brandon Reeder, Dimitri Svistunenko, Peter Nicholls and Mike Wilson.

References

1 Babcock GT, Wikstršm M. Oxygen activation and the conservation of energy in cell respiration. *Nature* 1992;**356**:301–9.

2 Alderton WK, Cooper CE, Knowles RG. Nitric oxide synthases: structure, function and inhibition. *Biochem J* 2001;**357**:593–615.

3 Kennedy JG, O'Grady P, McCarthy DR, *et al.* An investigation into the role of oxygen free radical scavengers in preventing polymethylmethacrylate-induced necrosis in an osteoblast cell culture. *Orthopedics* 2000;**23**:481–5.

4 Cooper CE. Ferryl iron and protein free radicals. In: Rice-Evans CA, Burdon RH, eds. *Free Radical Damage and its Control.* Amsterdam: Elsevier 1994, 65–109.

5 Alayash AI, Patel RP, Cashon RE. Redox reactions of hemoglobin and myoglobin: biological and toxicological implications. *Antioxid Redox Signal* 2001;**3**:313–27.

6 Svistunenko DA, Patel RP, Voloshchenko SV, Wilson MT. The globin-based free radical of ferryl hemoglobin is detected in normal human blood. *J Biol Chem* 1997;**272**:7114–21.

7 Holt SGR, Moore K. Pathogenesis of renal failure in rhabdomyolysis: the role of myoglobin. *Exp Nephrol* 2000;**8**:72–6.

8 Alayash AI. Hemoglobin-based blood substitutes and the hazards of blood radicals. *Free Rad Res* 2000;**33**:341–8.

9 Holt SGR. Rhabdomyolysis. In: Galley HF, ed. *Critical Care Focus, Volume 1: Renal Failure.* London: BMJ Books/Intensive Care Society 1999, 15–20.

10 Moore KP, Holt S, Patel RP, *et al.* A causative role for redox cycling of myoglobin and its inhibition by alkalinization in the pathogenesis and treatment of rhabdomyolysis-induced renal failure. *J Biol Chem* 1998;**273**:31731–7.

11 Holt S, Reeder B, Wilson M, *et al.* Increased lipid peroxidation in patients with rhabdomyolysis. *Lancet* 1999;**353**:1241.

12 Reeder BJ, Wilson MT. The effects of pH on the mechanism of hydrogen peroxide and lipid hydroperoxide consumption by myoglobin: a role for the protonated ferryl species. *Free Rad Biol Med* 2001;**30**:1311–18.

13 Sanders KE, Ackers G, Sligar S. Engineering and design of blood substitutes. *Curr Opin Struct Biol* 1996;**6**:534–40.

14 Winslow RM. Alpha-alpha-crosslinked hemoglobin: was failure predicted by preclinical testing? *Vox Sang* 2000;**79**:1–20.

15 D'Agnillo F, Alayash AI. Site-specific modifications and toxicity of blood substitutes. The case of diaspirin cross-linked hemoglobin. *Adv Drug Deliv Rev* 2000;**40**:199–212.

16 Dunne J, Svistunenko DA, Alayash AI, Wilson MT, Cooper CE. Reactions of cross-linked methaemoglobins with hydrogen peroxide. *Adv Exp Med Biol* 1999;**471**:9–15.

17 Privalle C, Talarico T, Keng T, DeAngelo J. Pyridoxalated hemoglobin polyoxyethylene: a nitric oxide scavenger with antioxidant activity for the treatment of nitric oxide-induced shock. *Free Rad Biol Med* 2000;**28**:1507–17.

18 Eich RF, Li TS, Lemon DD, *et al.* Mechanism of NO-induced oxidation of myoglobin and hemoglobin. *Biochemistry* 1996;**35**:6976–83.
19 Gross SS, Lane P. Physiological reactions of nitric oxide and hemoglobin: a radical rethink. *Proc Natl Acad Sci USA* 1999;**96**:9967–9.
20 Doherty DH, Doyle MP, Curry SR, *et al.* Rate of reaction with nitric oxide determines the hypertensive effect of cell-free hemoglobin. *Nat Biotechnol* 1998;**16**:672–6.
21 Rioux F, Harvey N, Moisan S, *et al.* Nonpeptide endothelin receptor antagonists attenuate the pressor effect of diaspirin-crosslinked hemoglobin in rat. *Can J Physiol Pharmacol* 1999;**77**:188–94.
22 Fischer SR, Traber DL. L-arginine and endothelin receptor antagonist bosentan counteract hemodynamic effects of modified hemoglobin. *Shock* 1999;**11**:283–90.
23 Jia L, Bonaventura C, Bonaventura J, Stamler JS. S-Nitrosohemoglobin – a dynamic activity of blood involved in vascular control. *Nature* 1996;**380**:221–6.

Index

Page numbers in **bold** type refer to figures; those in *italic* refer to tables or boxed material